FOOD GLORIOUS FOOD!

FOOD GLORIOUS FOOD!

Transcending Obesity through the Symbology of Freud and Jung

Written by
Nadine Jacobs

AEON

First edition published in 2022 by
Aeon Books

British Library Cataloguing in Publication Data

A C.I.P. for this book is available from the British Library

ISBN-13: 978-1-80152-026-3

Typeset by Medlar Publishing Solutions Pvt Ltd, India
Printed in Great Britain

www.aeonbooks.co.uk

CONTENTS

FOREWORD

Food glorious food!

In the last century food has become a multibillion-pound industry, food factories are printing money, and cooking programmes on television are currently more popular than soaps.

The result: our world population is becoming fatter and fatter.

More food is being produced now than ever before.

Modern-day gluttony has become daily ritual and despite the fact that obesity has captured global attention, public health systems are still increasingly under pressure. The cost of caring for people with lifestyle diseases typically associated with obesity, including diabetes, hypertension, and heart problems is an increasing problem in many countries.

Regardless of the staggering global statistics from the World Health Organization in 2015, reporting that 1.9 billion adults were overweight, of whom 600 million were obese, the same issue remains today. The reality is that year on year millions of people attempt to lose the weight that they have gained during their honeymoon, after giving birth, or after overindulgence during the festive season. Regardless of the reason, if you are reading this book, the chances are that you yourself have had a few failed attempts at losing those few extra pounds or unwanted belly fat. First, your failed attempts are not unique, most overweight or obese people have had multiple failed attempts. Second, statistics show that only two to five per cent of people who have lost weight success-fully manage to retain the weight loss over the long term. Despite the increasing availability of effective nutritional strategies, physical exer-cise regimes, and behaviour modification approaches to weight loss, none of these offer a satisfactory explanation as to why such low num-bers of people who have successfully lost weight, manage to keep it off or why obesity continues to rise.

In attempting to understand the complexity of these food patholo-gies, especially obesity, I am going to explore several concepts. First, where the importance of food comes from, that is, what foods have symbolised through history; and second, as it is not only its physical consumption that drives us to obesity, what else is there about food that drives us to consumption of food beyond the point of satiety?

In order to explore this symbolic meaning of food, its influence on conscious behaviour, and how it developed through history and across cultures, in order to discover the root of obesity, the book will be divided into five parts:

a. Exploring the narratives that have been conveyed through tradi-tions relating to food, in search of the symbolic meanings that are the unconscious root of people's dietary behaviour.
b. Determining the origins of symbolic meaning that people attach to food, by comparing food narratives over time.
c. Discovering cultural symbols that have become part of the uncon-scious narrative and how it has affected people's food consumption patterns.
d. Finding the link between the symbolic meaning of food and obesity.
e. Exploring how the unconscious influence of food symbols induces conscious dietary behaviour.

By discovering the link between unconscious symbols of food and food pathologies, perhaps these pathologies, especially obesity, can be tack-led and solved with greater success.

AN OVERVIEW OF THE BOOK

The chapter following describes the rationale for the book as filling a gap in the prevailing approaches to obesity; all of these lead to successful weight loss, and the validity of the prevailing dietary, nutritional, exercise, and behaviour modification approaches to treatment of obesity are not questioned. However, despite the significant weight loss achieved by means of these approaches, the statistics show that in the majority of cases, the weight loss is not sustained over the long run, as discovered by researchers Goodrick and Foreyt in 1991. Consequently, we need to turn to the unconscious and specifically the symbolic meaning the unconscious attaches to food and eating behaviour as a possible explanation for the failure to sustain long-term weight loss.

Chapter Two will start with a review of some of the literature and psychological approaches to obesity that are offered. The boundary and dysregulation model of obesity, as well as different theories of obesity will be explained. The importance of traditional models of obesity will also be highlighted in this chapter.

Chapter Three discusses the theoretical framework on which the book is grounded, namely the psychoanalytic approach that will be based on the contributions of Sigmund Freud and Carl Gustav Jung.

Thereafter, the work of Freud related to obesity will be explored, also discussing the literature contributions of Hilde Bruch as an example of applying the Freudian theory. It is followed by the Jungian approach to obesity, explaining the fundamental role that complexes and archetypes have on the unconscious. Comparisons and differences between the two theories will be highlighted throughout the chapter, in order to explain the significance of the psychoanalytic theory on food pathology. In this context, reference is made to the work of Marion Woodman.

Chapter Four explains the five concepts on which the book is based, namely symbols, food, obesity, the collective unconscious, and the personal unconscious. The chapter begins with an exploration of symbols and the significance that symbols have, and how symbols manifest in the unconscious and influence conscious behaviour. The second concept of food discusses the food symbols and myths of ancient time, and how these have changed through history. The power dynamics associated with food and its consumption are also extensively explored, as well as the prevailing medical opinion of obesity at different times in history. Similarly, food and the sharp focus on obesity, in particular in the current period of history, are illustrated with reference to body image and socio-economic class.

A further analysis of Jungian dynamics is explored during the fourth chapter of the book. Its starting point is to consider the impacts of recent advances in other fields, including quantum physics and bioelectronics, on the validity of Carl Jung's concept of the collective unconscious and the interconnectedness between the physical and mental worlds and the unconscious. The insights offered by quantum physics explain Jung's archetypes as wave forms existing in a quantum state of potentiality in the cosmic mind that can and do translate to matter in the empirical world. In particular, the impact of wave forms on the expression of cellular genetics provided by bioelectronics offers support to Marion Woodman who argued that the difference in the size of fat cells between obese and normal weight patients derive from their psyche, in particular the unconscious, which she further illustrates by exploring the complexes through a word association test devised by Jung. The differences between the Freudian and Jungian approaches are further illustrated in more depth and an application to the problem of obesity is offered through a further exploration of the archetypes.

The Alice texts of Lewis Carroll were selected to further illustrate the application of both approaches. Given the nature of the Alice texts, the anima/animus is explored in the Jungian reading of the text against the metaphor of the Hero's Journey of transformation towards individuation. In this reading, Alice is analysed as a character in the Jungian tradition of reading the dream as an act employed by the psyche to compensate for an imbalance in the psyche; in this case in the anima as represented by the Death Mother archetype.

The Freudian reading of the text focuses the analysis on the author Lewis Carroll and sees the dream as expressing repressed trauma on the part of the author. In particular, the Eros/Thanatos complex is explored. In Carroll's case, according to the highly sexualised Freudian reading of the text, the Eros/Thanatos imbalance translated in the occurrence of the *vagina dentata* as represented by Carroll's fear of the aggressive feminine represented by adult women and his ideation of little girls.

The final chapters offer a synthesis of the themes explored throughout the book before presenting the final concluding arguments, findings, and suggestions for further research. In addition, the last chapter offers the author's evaluation of the extent to which the research aim and objectives were met, as well as a consideration of the limitations presented by the scope and methodology employed in support of the book.

CHAPTER 1

The big O-word: obesity

Obesity is still today being stigmatised by most societies. Children are being bullied at school for being overweight and career opportunities are fewer for obese people. Obesity is a disease that is dreaded: an epidemic that affects and destroys all normality for the people suffering from it. Many of you reading this book can relate to the following scenarios to explain the term obesity. Obesity is that moment when you are sitting on a creaking, dainty glass-look-alike chair at a fancy gala dinner or a wedding, wondering if the chair is going to collapse under you at any minute. You try to "sit lighter" on it in order to prevent any possible embarrassment of breakage. Obesity is not fitting into any decent piece of clothing that your usual clothing store has to offer and eventually walking out of the shop with the one and only piece of clothing that remotely fits you. Later, when you look at yourself in the mirror wearing your new purchase of trousers, shirt, or dress, you realise that you now look like a fine replica of the rent-a-tent advertisement, the only difference is your tent has a face, hands, and feet. As obesity is a global issue, an endless number of studies have been conducted to discover the core of the issue. In this chapter we will look at some of the results of both successful and unsuccessful studies of weight loss and how they link to the global issue of obesity.

Studies have proven that the onset of obesity in both children and adults is alike and is a combination of reduced physical activities and bad eating habits, as depicted by William Dietz in 1983, but the psychology of changing these habits is not yet fully understood.

Literature and psychological approaches to obesity: sustainability and successful long-term weight loss = limited successful results

With obesity rates that have doubled in less than three decades (between 1980 and 2008), obesity has become a global issue that seeks treatment proposals and, more importantly, solutions (Grebitus, Hartmann, & Reynolds, 2015; Nurkkala et al., 2015). The World Health Organization (WHO) estimated that approximately 35 per cent of adults were overweight and a further 12 per cent were obese (WHO, 2004 as cited in Grebitus et al., 2015). Yet, there are no confirmed records of successful public health interventions that have yielded sustainable long-term weight loss or resulted in the successful reduction in obesity rates in populations (Hafekost, Lawrence, Mitrou, O'Sullivan, & Zubrick, 2013).

Dissonance in the holistic approach to combat obesity

Katherine Hafekost and her associates have studied twenty-seven articles that were written in 2011 on weight loss interventions and concluded that there is dissonance between the physiologic rudiments of weight loss/gain and interventions to address the prevalence of obesity in populations. They stated that there is a lack of collaboration on multidisciplinary levels and due to a lack of understanding of basic science behind weight loss interventions. The lack of collaboration leads to unfitting research questions being asked; hence no concrete solutions are found to the pressing issue of increasing rates of obesity. Hafekost and associates concluded that the approach to weight loss interventions should be multidisciplinary and should be based on biologically credible mechanisms.

The association of high-density lipoprotein cholesterol (HDLC) escalation and reduced visceral abdominal fat after weight loss intervention

Many studies have associated weight loss (even short-term intervention) with reduced risk of metabolic disorders such as hypertension, cardiovascular disease, and irregular levels of lipids or glucose in the blood. With the risk of regaining weight after weight loss in mind, Matsuo and his colleagues (2010) concentrated on metabolic risk factors that have an effect on the maintenance of long-term weight loss. The results were inconclusive. The study included dietary adaptations, exercise programmes, and counselling sessions by qualified dieticians. The results showed an improvement of risk factors during the initial fourteen-week period, however the risk factors rotated back to the point of departure after 105 weeks, regardless of the participants' maintenance of reduced visceral abdominal fat and mean body weight. Their study also succeeded in maintaining long-term weight loss; regardless of the fact that there was a slight increase during week 14 and 105. They established a positive relationship between visceral abdominal fat and HDLC, in that reduced visceral fat accompanies improvements on HDLC, but warned that it might also be influenced by hormone levels, which required further study. They also expressed their need for additional studies in understanding the link between dietary values and variations in metabolic risk factors.

Counselling on eating behaviour as a lifestyle intervention

Regardless of many studies that have been conducted to determine effective methods to achieve weight loss, an unflawed and effective weight loss method has not yet been determined. Marjukka Nurkkala and associates (2015) conducted an intensive lifestyle counselling intervention programme over three years, during which they investigated the influence of the eating behaviours of seventy-six subjects. They compared eating behaviours (cognitive restraint of eating, unrestrained eating, and responsive eating) to motivation to lose weight and tolerance to weight loss difficulties or challenges. The authors found that:

1. Healthy eating habits and regular physical activity, correlated with nutritional counselling, does result in weight loss, weight maintenance, and in some cases changes in nutritional habits (Andrade et al., 2010; Dombrowski, Knittle, Avenell, Araujo-Soares, & Sniehotta, 2014; Rejeski, Mihalko, Ambrosius, Bearon, & McClelland, 2011).
2. Implementing higher cognitive restraints enhances weight loss (Andrade et al., 2010; Keränen et al., 2009; Svendsen et al., 2008; Westerterp-Plantenga, Kempen, & Saris, 1998).

3. Personality types that are associated with binge eating and unrestrained eating, seldom display successful weight loss results and maintenance (Keränen et al., 2009; Pacanowski, Senso, Oriogun, Crain, & Sherwood, 2014; Svendsen et al., 2008; Westerterp-Plantenga, Kempen, & Saris, 1998).
4. Successful dieters are more effective in cognitive restraint from eating, than those who eat uncontrollably and do not stick to their diet (Karhunen et al., 2012; Keränen et al., 2009; Neve, Morgan, & Collins, 2012).
5. Also, people with higher body mass were inclined to show decreased levels of cognitive restraint (De Lauzon et al., 2004).

Nurkkala and colleagues emphasised that although a significant correlation between eating behaviour and successful weight loss has been established, there were very few studies that highlighted the effects of change in eating behaviour during long-term interventions. They concluded that self-confidence, motivation, self-efficacy, and the belief that one can change one's eating behaviour, are very important in successful weight loss and are not dependent on short-term or long-term counselling according to Anna-Maria Keränen and associates. Deborah Riebe and her associates (2005) also concluded that people with higher self-efficacy were better able to maintain their weight, more successful in weight loss, experienced less weight loss relapses, tended to exercise regularly, and could decline unhealthy food more easily.

In another study related to self-efficacy, Martin Teufel and associates similarly hypothesised in 2013 that behavioural changes can take place once self-efficacy has improved. They explained that people with obesity are confronted with two problems: "(1) Eating often serves as a dysfunctional relaxation technique in the absence of other stress-management skills; (2) Eating and food become individual stressors themselves because of negative consequences in emotion and cognition (frustration, shame, all-or-nothing thinking, etc.)." A food-specific bio-feedback model was developed that examined electro dermal activity of thirty-one women. Variables such as self-efficacy, stress levels, relaxation abilities, and dietary behaviour were also assessed prior, during, and three months after the assessment. Like the first mentioned study, the authors also concluded that improved self-efficacy, stress relieving, and relaxation mechanisms were associated with improved behavioural intentions and reduced psychological burden. A longitudinal study was necessary to confirm the results, as factors such as blood glucose and satiety were not taken into account.

After researching numerous articles on obesity and treatment of obesity, there are four main issues that were prevalent in these studies:

1. A holistic approach to obesity is inevitable. A successful model will have to include input from different disciplines (Baranowski, Cullen, Nicklas, Thompson, & Baranowski, 2003; Bea & Lohman, 2010; Drieling, Rosas, Ma, & Stafford, 2014; Grebitus, Hartmann, & Reynolds, 2015; Hafekost, Lawrence, Mitrou, O'Sullivan, & Zubrick, 2013; Legenbauer, Petrak, de Zwaan, & Herpertz, 2011; Martinez et al., 2016; Petek, Kern, Kovač-Blaž, & Kersnik, 2011; Teufel et al., 2013; Yeh, Chu, Hsu, Hsu, & Chung, 2015).
2. Behavioural change is necessary in order to attain long-term weight loss (Baranowski, Cullen, Nicklas, Thompson, & Baranowski, 2003; Martinez et al., 2016; Nurkala et al., 2015; Teufel et al., 2013).
3. Self-efficacy plays an important role in weight loss and obesity, as obesity is linked to low self-efficacy (Baranowski, Cullen, Nicklas, Thompson, & Baranowski, 2003; Grebitus, Hartmann, & Reynolds, 2015; Martinez et al., 2016; Nurkkala et al., 2015; Teufel et al., 2013).
4. Longitudinal studies and/or larger sample sizes are needed to determine the success of existing models that address obesity (Bea & Lohman, 2010; Drieling, Rosas, Ma, & Stafford, 2014; Legenbauer, Petrak, de Zwaan, & Herpertz, 2011; Martinez et al., 2016; Matsuo et al., 2010; Nurkkala et al., 2015; Petek, Kern, Kovač-Blaž, & Kersnik, 2011; Teufel et al., 2013; Yeh, Chu, Hsu, Hsu, & Chung, 2015).

For many patients, a last resort is to turn to surgical weight reduction treatment, such as bariatric surgery. Unfortunately, the success rate of this radical weight loss measure is not 100 per cent. A failure rate of 20 per cent has been reported by Tanja Legenbauer and associates (2011), with patients who fail to maintain a healthy BMI or those who regain weight after the surgery and initial weight loss. They concluded that most dieters, in general, return back to the weight they were before they started, and explained that in morbidly obese patients with a BMI that is higher than 40 kg/m^2, non-surgical weight loss proves to be so ineffective that bariatric surgery is becoming a recommended option for these patients to lose weight.

Given the link between self-efficacy and successful weight loss, the psychological origin of the lack of self-efficacy on moderating eating behaviour is relevant.

Traditional models of obesity

Overriding internal food cues: the boundary and dysregulation models

David Schlundt and his fellow researchers observed in 1991 that people with obesity tend to alternate periods of healthy eating habits and strict food intake restraint with periods of uncontrolled eating, and in many cases episodic binge eating, revealing the complexity of obese and overweight people's eating patterns.

The behavioural mechanism underlying these alternating eating patterns is the topic of several theories, with the majority focusing on dysfunctional behaviour. Janet Polivy and Peter Herman's (1987) boundary model seeks to explain patterns of overeating among adults and children by noting that it is impossible to maintain an energy restrictive diet constantly, and that attempts to do so over an extended period eventually leads to relapse when the dieter succumbs to episodes of uncontrolled binge eating.

The model further points out that repeated attempts to stick to energy restrictive dietary regimes produces another consequence: the biological limits of hunger and satiety are moved over time and are replaced with a cognitive limit instead, therefore the chances of failure increases if this self-imposed regulation is put to the test when the dieter is emotional. The dysregulation model of obesity, proposed by Gillian O'Reilly and associates (2014), similarly explains that as episodes of extreme energy restriction alternate with episodes of uncontrolled and binge eating, the natural satiety and hunger stimuli are overridden and eventually weaken to the point where these are no longer heeded, fuelling further episodes of overeating.

The inability to recognise hunger and satiety develops through three maladaptive cycles that tend to occur in the binge eater's life which cause an eventual delay in the response to hunger and satiety cues. Linda Craighead and Heather Allen describe these cycles as:

The dieting cycle. As illustrated in Figure 1, adapted from Christopher Fairburn, Terence Wilson, and K. Schleimer's model (1993), the dieting cycle starts when a person on diet consciously ignores hunger cues. In turn, as the hunger escalates, the person eventually gives in and ends up overeating as they disregard the body's response in the form of moderate internal satiety cues. In response to the binge eating, the dieter often faces extreme regret about the loss of self-control and tends to engage in negative self-talk, which triggers the *abstinence violation effect (AVE)*—a psychological term for violating personal boundaries that one sets for oneself. The Abstinence Violation Effect usually is followed by the *negative affect cycle* which tends to lead to the dieter adopting a harsher diet plan to compensate for the binge.

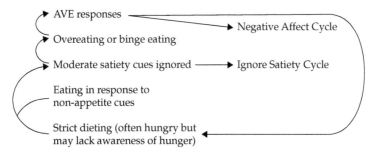

Figure 1: The dieting cycle (Craighead & Allen, 1996, p. 257).

The negative affect cycle. This particular cycle serves as an immediate but temporary relief and "reinforces food as a coping response for negative affect" (Craighead & Allen, 1996, p. 257). This cycle is explained in Figure 2.

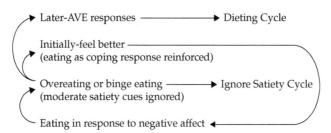

Figure 2: The negative affect cycle (Craighead & Allen, 1996, p. 257).

Unsurprisingly, as the dieting and negative affect cycles are repeated, the *ignore satiety cycle* develops (see Figure 3). Another origin of the ignore satiety cycle arises from environmental cues, such as regimented meal times which may not coincide with hunger, leading to a situation where people are conditioned to eat at certain times irrespective of hunger, and this requires them to ignore satiety.

The ignore satiety cycle. As binge eaters' sensitivity to satiety cues weakens, they arrive at a point where they will only stop eating when these signals become quite strong and manifest as the discomfort associated with overeating. This is the AVE which is when the initial satiety cues are ignored and the binge eater will only stop eating in the presence of an environmental factor (such as an empty plate) or when discomfort sets in as a result of overeating.

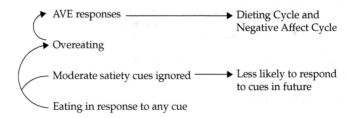

Figure 3: The ignore satiety cycle (Craighead & Allen, 1996, p. 258).

According to Craighead and Allen, these cycles can be broken through appetite awareness training which helps binge eaters to identify satiety cues so that they can prevent binge eating.

While the boundary model, and the dysregulation model that followed it, mainly explains bulimia nervosa, according to Fairburn and associates, its explanatory ability falls short in that it does not adequately explain the eating problems of people with obesity. For instance, approximately half of the people with obesity quoted in a 1997 study by Spurrell, Wilfley, Tanofsky, and Brownell reported that their first episode of binge eating preceded their first diet. It therefore suggests that in order to fully grasp the essence of the problem it would be prudent to distinguish between the people with obesity who have repeated episodes of binge eating and those who do not and, similarly, to distinguish between people who have followed energy restrictive diets and those who have not.

The externality theory. Another theoretical suggestion is that the personality of the obese person may explain the propensity towards obesity; particularly insofar as impulse control is concerned, as explained by Boutelle and associates in 2014. The externality theory suggests that obese and overweight people are "external eaters", noting that externality is a personality trait. Obese and overweight people tend to exhibit higher trait impulsiveness and consequently are also more likely to engage in other impulsive behavioural patterns including substance abuse, according to Douglas Chalmers, Chester Bowyer, and Nancy Olenick (1990). Externality theory holds that people with obesity tend to display an increased responsiveness (i.e. immediate eating) towards food triggered by external cues including taste, smell, and appearance, and that these external cues override internal cues such as satiety, but the theory was subject to intense criticism in that with respect to obesity the externality theory did not demonstrate causality or sufficient universality.

While people with obesity admittedly do show a greater responsiveness to external food cues, Caroline Braet and Tatjana Van Strien (1997) state that the precursor remains unclear insofar as uncertainty remains on whether the heightened response to external food cues determines the onset of obesity or whether the obesity causes the heightened sensitivity to external food cues. Following from the notion that a person's reaction to external stimuli, such as food, is learned behaviour, it follows that this behaviour can be unlearned through conditioning. Boutelle and his associates sought to inhibit the response to external sensory stimuli by altering response behaviour to respond more effectively to hunger and satiety, resulting in fewer tendencies to overeat.

To achieve this, Braet and Van Strien developed two different treatments, targeting obese children. First, the "Children's Appetite Awareness" training sought to strengthen their sensitivity to hunger and satiety cues which would allow them to improve their eating habits. Second, the "Cue Exposure Treatment" targeted the eating behaviour of children when they have already reached a moderate level of satiety. In this case the treatment sought to decrease the children's reaction to hunger cues so that they could reduce their food consumption. The treatments were combined with self-monitoring exercises, parenting assistance, and coping skills training. Their study showed that children's reaction to hunger and satiety cues could be moderated through effective treatment and education, but more studies needed to be done to determine the success rate on adults.

Caroline Braet and Geert Crombez (2003) also found that these and similar therapeutic approaches that were aimed at reducing the responsiveness to external food cues have been successful. Where hypersensitivity to food cues exists in a patient, it was found that this information bias tends to initiate dysfunctional eating behaviour. Consequently, information processing mechanisms, specifically hypersensitivity to food cues, are now regarded as an alternative explanation for obese children's inability to resist external food cues.

The learning theory. In contrast, pointing to learning theories of behaviour, C. Ferster, C. J. Nurenburger, and Alexandra Levitt (1962) posit that the immediate enjoyment and satiety impact the eating behaviour and tend to override it in the long term, often with the negative consequences of weight gain. In other words, people with obesity have learned bad eating habits. This theory explains why bad eating habits persist despite the obese person fully appreciating the long-term negative consequences. Further, the theory also noted that people tend to eat more, out of habit, when emotionally distressed (as a learned response), and when distracted (e.g. eating while watching television).

One response to absent-minded eating is to introduce mindful eating, in that mindfulness "as a quality of consciousness that is characterised by optimally attending to one's moment-by-moment experiences, thoughts, and emotions with an open and non-judgmental approach" (O'Reilly, Cook, Spruijt-Metz, & Black, 2014, p. 2), can improve emotional and sensory awareness; and as a consequence, could improve self-control. The learning theory goes further, to contend that as people eat in different situations, different stimuli become associated with food, forming powerful associations. Hence the therapeutic approach should seek to reduce the situations as this in turn reduces the associative value of the external stimuli—in other words, unlearning the eating behaviour by unlearning the associations.

Paul Karoly and Frederick Kanfer (1982) hold that self-regulation exercises, combined with a sharp reduction in the number of eating situations, and focusing on elements such as the development of problem-solving techniques, are all elements of weight loss therapy based on the learning approach. While according to Terence Wilson (1994), deficiencies in problem-solving ability had been observed in obese children, the learning theory falls short in that it does not distinguish the conditions facilitating the learning of bad eating behaviour from those that do not, and while the learning theory underpins the majority of programmes offered to obese children, the theory itself is still in need of further evaluation and refinement.

For Richard Ganley (1996), the family context is also considered in the onset and development of obesity, particularly in children, in that food is often used as a way to reinforce or punish behaviour. Leann Birch (1987) explained that the food used as a reward (typically sweets for children) consequently becomes more attractive in general (see also Boakes, Popplewell, & Burton, 1987), whereas the family context also explains other learned eating behaviour such as finishing the food on one's plate, the tolerance of hunger, dealing with frustrations, and resisting food impulses (Johnson & Birch, 1994). In this context, the inability to control eating behaviour is seen as an indicator of a broader behavioural problem, as children who have not learned control over their eating habits may also encounter a general lack of self-control. This in turn implies that any behavioural therapy seeking to overcome this inability to self-regulate may have to address the parenting skills as well. Child obesity can thus be seen as a function of a family pathology, according to Hilde Bruch (1973).

Bruch also made additional observations in 1973 about obese family members in that they have weak boundaries between subsystems and also little autonomy, yet clinical case studies specifically focusing on measuring family interactions are scarce due to the difficulties in observing family interactions. Yet Heather Banis and her associates (1988), as well as Beverley Mendelson and Donna White (1995) noted that obese families tend to exhibit less cohesion and a more authoritarian approach to parenting than non-obese families. Joop Bosch, Margreet Stradmeijer, and Jaap Seidell (2004) found that non-obese families tend to favour a more democratic approach to child rearing, while the interactions in obese families are more hostile and parents with obese children are more likely to openly reject them. However, these studies are not conclusive as they were mainly cross-sectional. Longitudinal studies are thus required to establish the extent to which a dysfunctional family context (including ineffective parenting) contributes to the onset and development of pathology in the form of eating disorders; particularly obesity, according to Braet and Van Strien (1997).

The psycho-symptomatic theory. The psycho-symptomatic theory of obesity, put forward by Wendy Wallace, Dave Sheslow, and Sandy Hassink (1993), suggests that people with obesity tend to cope with negative feelings by eating and the reason why people with obesity eat more than others is because of the inability to distinguish hunger from emotional arousal. However, David Allison and Stanley Heshka (1993) found insufficient evidence to sustain this proposition, in that the link between obesity and emotional eating is not strong enough to imply causality.

Braet and Van Strien (1997) as well as Albert Stunkard and Jeffery Sobal (1995) found, however, that people with obesity remain exposed to various psychological impacts arising from their obesity given prevailing social attitudes, which tend to reject people with obesity based on their appearance. This, in turn, affects the way people with obesity relate socially, and people with obesity tend to feel less loved and are more likely to be subjected to teasing and social scorn according to Cyd Strauss and associates in 1985. However, research on self-image issues arising from obesity needs further refinement in that these studies do not distinguish between those who are obese and those who are merely overweight; differences attributable to age or gender; and the heterogeneity of samples, according to Beverly Mendelson and Donna White (1985).

Stuart Fine, Glenn Haley, Mervyn Gilbert, and Adele Forth (1993) stated similarly that the prevailing research is inconclusive as to whether the problems associated with obesity tend to increase linearly or parallel with the increase in weight. Wendy Wallace and her associates (1993) also stated that while the occurrence of childhood and depression is noted, this co-morbidity has not been shown to imply causality.

The importance of the traditional models of obesity explained

The four theories that have been discussed seem to point towards overeating as a result of either the inability to recognise an internal cue (the dieting cycle theory), or responding to the wrong cue (the externality theory), or mistaking the cue for something else and responding inappropriately (the psychosomatic theory) which points to maladaptive responses to mental and physical signals, resulting in problematic eating behaviour. The remedy proposed in all four theories suggests a redirection of the focus of those who are overweight, either through learning to recognise satiety cues, de-emphasising external stimuli in favour of internal satiety cues, or by recognising the emotional cues and correcting the response. Thus, weight loss, although greatly aided by reduced energy intake and exercise, cannot be sustained in the absence of a psychological intervention that seeks to introduce mindfulness to eating behaviour. Mindfulness is a "quality of consciousness that is characterised by continually attending to one's moment-by-moment experiences, thoughts and emotions with an open, non-judgmental approach" (O'Reilly, Cook, Spruijt-Metz, & Black, 2014, p. 2). The effective and conscious practice of mindfulness improves emotional and sensory awareness and consequently improves self-control.

Nevertheless, while the introduction of mindfulness in weight loss therapy holds promise, the authors point out that it remains a complementary therapy which needs to be supplemented by those factors that enable an individual to successfully initiate and sustain lifestyle changes. These include self-efficacy, goal-oriented behaviour, social support and other motivational factors, incremental and actual goal attainment, and previous behaviour patterns. Ingela Kvalem and associates (2016) identified the ability to self-regulate and control impulsive behaviour as a key factor in maintaining long-term weight loss and an important predictor in the ultimate success of patients who sought bariatric surgery. They define self-regulation as having control over the thoughts and focus of attention that ultimately affects one's behaviour. The ability to reflect on one's self, through self-observation and reflection on past behaviour, underpins one's ability to learn from experience and this, with self-efficacy, underpins the self-regulating process. Consistent self-regulation, motivation for change, clear goals, and a solid expectation of weight loss are a few recommendations they suggest for making successful lifestyle changes.

CHAPTER 2

Psychoanalytic theories of Sigmund Freud and Carl Jung

The problem with Jung's work, as I have gathered through the years on the lonely planet of Jungians, is that his work is so complex and rich in information that few people will bother to understand it.

A friend of mine once asked me about my master's thesis in 2017 and as I started explaining to her that I used Jung's theories to discover the root of obesity, she asked me, "Who is Jung?" But the next moment she answered her own question and said: "Oh yes! I saw the movie of Jung and Freud! That guy was not right in the head hey … sex, sex, sex and sex!" She referred to the movie *The Dangerous Method* that was released in 2011. While changing to a closed position in crossing her arms and legs in her chair, looking at me from the side of her eye with a raised eyebrow, she said, "What did you find?", with a very distrusting tone in her voice.

Immediately I had an Ally McBeal moment (for those of you who do not know, *Ally McBeal* was a comedy show in the 1990s of a woman in a very ordinary office job with an extraordinary imagination) that took me right back to my first year of BA psychology when we were learning about the different original theorists of psychology. On this day the discussion on Jung followed after the discussion of Freud. The lecturer introduced the theorist Jung with "… which brings us to eeky freeky Jung". I found her comment rather invective and till this day I recall her as a little girl with pigtails and putting her thumbs in her ears, waving her hands forwards and backwards as if they were giant elephant ears, putting her face very close to mine, singing in a nagging voice: "Eeky freaky Jung! Eeky freaky Jung! Eeky freaky Jung."

Having read many books and articles on Jung before I started studying psychology, it will be an understatement to say that I was bitterly insulted as a first-year student on that day. After I completed the dissertation for my master's degree, we became friends and I still tease her today about "eeky freeky Jung". Instead of introducing Jung as "eeky freeky Jung", she now gives students an assignment to make an appointment with a Jungian in order to gather information on the theorist Carl Gustaf Jung. Upon which prompt I regularly get an email a few days later from a group of students who want to interview me on the personality theory of Jung. I always gladly accept and when the students (usually between five and eight of them) are all crammed in my little 25 square metre office, some sitting on chairs, some sitting on the floor, and usually one or two sitting very uncomfortably with one buttock on my desk. They always struggle to hide their initial disappointment when I say: "Well, about his work on personality theory I cannot tell you much, as Jung himself said that his personality theory is some of his earliest and most basic work on which people measured his ability and neglected to see his profound and meaningful work later, such as the collective unconscious." Immediately, their thoughts of "this is going to be an easy assignment" blow up in thin air as part of the assignment is about the personality theory of Jung.

But then, to soothe their disappointment, I would say to them in an enticing voice: "So, if you want to hear more about his profound work on the collective unconscious, complexes, archetypes, symbols in fairy tales and dreams, then I can help you." And usually their eyes would become interested, they would settle in like pre-schoolers ready to listen to a story that the kindergarten teacher is going to read on the carpet in their classroom, sitting cross-legged and excitingly turning their heads towards the teacher's voice.

Then I start … What do you know about Jung? Archetypes? Symbols? The collective unconscious? Some group members would have done some research before they came and others would pretend to be invisible so that I would not consider looking in their direction or ask them a question.

I then explain to them what I know about these terms, give them examples, and let them apply the information to their own lives to make it easier to understand, and eventually they would leave very satisfied with the information I gave them, regardless that I did not answer their original question. And then there is always one student that stays behind unnoticed after all the other students have left. Usually, this one person was the quiet one in the group and he or she will ask some more questions about Jung or the applicability of Jung on his or her life and will always ask shyly towards the end of the meeting: "Ma'am, may I come again? I mean, just to talk more about Jung?"

Being a closet Jungian is not easy. My heart always warms for such students, because I know where they are in their lives. They understand so much more than their fellow classmates, but they do not dare to talk, because nobody understands them. In the land of sexy Freud, who wants to admit that they are actually followers of something more profound?, something phenomenal: Eeky freaky Jung.

It is my belief that some people who do not understand a concept will rather belittle it, instead of taking the time and making the effort to understand certain concepts. People do not want to admit for the fear of judgment that they do not know something and will rather laugh it off as irrelevant information.

When a person reads books written by Carl Jung, one has to really sit and think what he is saying, sit and analyse what he means. Many of his words you have to feel to understand what he is saying, and often this is where the problem with Jung comes in: in many ways we have to look at ourselves and at our own lives and experiences in order to understand Jung. People do not like to face themselves; people do not like to look at themselves in the mirror and see their issues and their shortcomings. Jung's work holds a mirror that reflects the deepest and darkest corners of our being, our lives, and our experiences.

I can only compare Jung's work with a power tool such as a mitre saw. If you do not know what you are doing you can cut off your fingers, or even your arm. But once you have mastered the art of using a mitre saw, you can create the most beautiful furniture, objects, and even houses.

If you are willing to look in the mirror of the unconscious that the Jungian theory holds up in front of you, you can explore the magnificent person that you are and you can learn to live with the scars of past trauma, without it destroying your future.

The chapter will thus focus on explaining and simplifying psychoanalytic approaches as proposed by Sigmund Freud and Carl Jung. These two approaches will be contrasted with each other to highlight the differences between Freud's and Jung's understanding of the human psyche and how they differed in their view on the manner in which the unconscious translates into conscious behaviour. Both Freud and Jung wrote extensively on the unconscious, yet they differed markedly in their understanding of its function in the psychological process. Where both Freud and Jung agreed on the existence of the personal unconscious, Jung took the concept further by postulating the existence of the collective unconscious. Given the scope of this book, both approaches are relevant in understanding how the complexes, archetypes, and symbols of the unconscious contribute to the onset and development of pathology in the form of eating disorders, particularly obesity.

The psychoanalytic theory and its importance explained

On balance, the contemporary theories of obesity converge on the central theme of the importance of self-efficacy in attaining and maintaining weight loss. What the contemporary theories do not explain is why some people, including those facing the disastrous and life threatening health consequences of morbid obesity, do not respond to the various approaches proposed to enhance self-efficacy. What these theoretical approaches share, however, is a focus on conscious behaviour and they all seek to intervene on the conscious level. The psychoanalytic approach presents a departure from the contemporary theories in that these theories suggest that conscious behaviours are largely the product of unconscious drives. Thus, to effect a lasting behavioural change, the roots of the pathological behaviour must be uncovered in the unconscious: a domain in the human psyche that is irrational and symbolic.

The psychoanalytic explanation of why some people do not respond to weight loss therapy, sustainably and in the long term (exceeding one year), would be that there are fundamental issues residing in the unconscious, which if left unaddressed, would consistently result in self-sabotage behaviour despite the best intent of the dieter. Put differently, the self-efficacy, so important in moderating eating behaviour and resulting in healthier lifestyle choices, would not be achieved without an intervention directed at the unconscious. Given the failure of weight loss interventions in achieving long-term and sustainable results in the face of very real adverse health consequences for those who do not succeed in losing and keeping the weight off, the theoretical lens adopted by this book is that presented by the psychoanalytic approaches of Freud and Jung; its focus on the unconscious, and given the symbolic nature and expression of the unconscious, the importance of food symbols in uncovering the unconscious drives of pathological eating behaviour.

The process of Freudian psychoanalysis was explained by Alan Spivak in 2014, as the excavation of impulses and reactions that were stored as symbols in the unconscious, but connected to an emotion or reaction in the conscious. Psychoanalysis is the tool to translate unconscious symbols back to conscious reactions and emotions, thus reversing the process as the symbol is used to recall or explore the underlying reaction or emotion that resulted in the symbol in the first place.

Through language, the patient can put into words what he or she feels. Freud advocated active feeling in the moment to enable the analysis of the impulse to be fully understood. The feeling is thus not experienced as an outsider, but it becomes reality for the client and the therapist resulting in the relief of the anxiety relating to unwillingness to listen to oneself, by bringing the unconscious reaction or emotion to the surface.

Spivak perceives words not only as the carriers of emotion, but also as symbols that are stored for impending reflection or internal exploration. Words thus become the powerful transferring tool when the client experiences conflicting emotions within. It is as if the symbols overflow, causing unsettling feelings in the unconscious, pushing it through to the conscious, where it can be acknowledged and analysed through psychoanalysis in its active stage. When these emotions have been acknowledged, translated, deconstructed, interpreted, the unconscious can be understood. The interpretation of the symbolic meaning in Freudian analysis is aimed at understanding the transference phenomenon, the compulsion behind the response as well as the defence reactions that it triggers. The analyst guides the client through exploration of emotions by using countertransference and empathetically tapping into the client's experiences and perceptions of his or her world. Through this, the analyst can experience the event subjectively as a person, but also objectively as the analyst.

The effective result of integration is the reduction of anxiety and the lowering of defences. The fear or negative emotion that has been attached to the symbol is now transformed and once again stored into the unconscious.

The psychoanalytic theory: Freud

The id, ego, and superego. Jung's early support of Freud derived from their shared interest in the unconscious. Freud saw the unconscious mind as the epicentre of repressed thoughts and traumatic memories and as the location of hidden sexual desires, which, because they are repressed, leads to neurosis. Freud proposed that the human psyche comprised three structures; the pleasure principle known as the *id*, which is not bound by morality, but instead seeks to achieve pleasure and forms unconscious energies (mainly sexual); it is influenced by the *superego* which seeks to moderate the impulses of the *id* into socially acceptable behaviour and the *ego* which comprises our conscious memories and thoughts.

Freud argued that the instincts originating in the *id* are the impulses of all behaviour and identified them as Eros (love) and the destructive or death instinct. The purpose of the love instinct is to form connections and to preserve unity through relationships with others. In contrast, the death instinct seeks to undo connections and unity through destruction. Freud further posited that these two instincts can operate either exclusively from each other, or combine through attraction.

The conscious, preconscious, and unconscious. Freud's view of the human psychological process distinguishes between the conscious, preconscious, and unconscious. In the conscious domain, one is aware of ideas, but only briefly, while preconscious ideas are ideas that are capable of becoming conscious, but are not yet conscious. Unconscious ideas are not easily accessible, but they can be inferred, recognised, and explained through analysis. Freud held that the unconscious thoughts of the *id* attempted to force their way into consciousness through dreams, which can originate either in the *id* or the *ego*. The dreams are characterised by their strong use of symbolism and are the product of conflict and have the power to either bring up memories the dreamer had forgotten or to bring up impressions which could not have originated from the dreamer's mind. Freud cautioned that what the individual recalls from the dream is only the façade behind which the meaning must be inferred.

Freud emphasised that "it is our impulses that are speaking and making us act" (Freud, 1900a, p. 73) and discussed the concept of transference as that which "provides the impulse necessary for understanding and translating the language of the unconscious; where it is lacking, the patient does not make the effort or does not listen when we submit our translation to him" (1900a, p. 11). Hence, people make meaning of experiences through unconscious translation and transference. Freud perceived the unconscious as a storage mechanism for the frightening and unknown "symptoms of transference" (1900a, p. 1064).

According to Werner Meyer, Cora Moore, and Henning Viljoen (2008), Freud noted that the suppression of unconscious thoughts, emotions, and memories is the defence mechanism that the ego deploys to protect itself from the real emotions and inner conflict that these events may produce.

Developmental stages. Freud defined several developmental stages commencing with the oral and anal gratification stages before moving to the more advanced stages. Freud's psychosexual development theory found its early application to the problem of obesity in the work of Hilde Bruch who noted common features in obese children including immaturity, overdependence, and a lack of aggressiveness. She suggested that the obese child tends to respond to traumatic experiences such as failure and disappointment by overeating as the "heavy layer of fat is like a wall behind which the child seeks protection against a hostile outside world" (Bruch, 1941, p. 467).

In terms of Freud's developmental stages, childhood obesity was seen as a fixation at the oral stage of psychosexual development as Gustav Bychowski noted in 1950: "In surrounding herself with a cushion of fat, she was unconsciously attempting to avoid her mother's wrath—since she was eliminating herself as a rival (Oedipus)—and her father's anger at her potential relations with other men" (Bruch, 1941, p. 327).

Jung rejected Freud's emphasis on the libido as primarily a sexual energy, arguing that instead it was a generalised psychic energy that served as a motivating force for the intellectual development, spirituality, and creativity of the individual. In particular, Jung explored the psychic energy as a general life force and motivational source for seeking pleasure and reducing conflict. In this, sexuality is but one manifestation of it, but certainly not the only one. Jung also vehemently disagreed with Freud's Oedipus and Electra theories, instead arguing that the early relationship between mother and child was based on the love and protection afforded by the mother to the child, an idea which was later further developed by John Bowlby and Mary Ainsworth in attachment theory and internal models (Ainsworth & Bowlby, 1991; Bretherton, 1992).

In her 2002 presentation of the psychodynamics of food and its consumption, Susanne Skubal illustrated that the act of eating is essentially an individual act, whether done in solitude or in a social context. Even in a social context most people still eat their individual portions together, but separately in that they each use their own plates. The fact remains that whether food consumption is done in isolation or in identifying and bonding with others in a social context, eating remains a life-affirming act.

Skubal noted that our first and last Eros remains oral, and in contrast to Freud, quotes psychoanalytic psychologist Karl Abraham who asserts that the psychological phenomenon connected to the genital zone is not as primary as those connected with the oral zone. Skubal took this concept further by noting that the consideration of orality must confront both the divided nature of eating (isolated or social) in addition to its doubled nature in that the mouth is both a locus of need and a satisfier of desire. In that, the mouth becomes the recurring site of lack (hunger) and loss (the experience of being weaned) as well as the place of pleasurable and sustainable recompense (nurture and nutrition). The dual nature of the mouth lies in it being both the place of ingestion and utterance. The mouth also becomes bilingual in that it speaks both the language of the father and mother. According to the creation myth of the Bible, in the beginning was the word, while for Freud, the beginning starts with a deed; food nourishes the body, but it also has meaning—and we remain with these mouths that can commit miracles or mayhem in both word and deed.

Skubal presents an analysis that starts with the trinity of human identity, memory, and mother, and describes how these are defined by the oral—in particular the oral bond that forms in infancy. Most of human existence starts with a simple script, as babies are born and take in the universe. She noted that to know biblically is to know sexually, but to know physically is to know orally. Therefore, the first months of an infant's life are defined around dependence on the mother for nourishment, through the child's mouth—this is human life. Skubal noted that nourishment/human life only occurs in the presence of another, which is either the breast or a surrogate. This makes the infant's life conditional upon the presence of the other, even before the infant's sight has developed fully and through the rooting reflex, the infant instinctively knows which way to turn to find the breast.

In this paradigm, the connection is the breast and the mouth, not only as a condition for physical survival, but upon this biological imperative the basis for all human connectedness is created, according to Skubal. Echoing the concept, British psychoanalyst John Bowlby further noted that the body intimacy that develops in the feeding embrace not only elicits a first, radical knowledge, but becomes the basis for the entire psychological and physiological development of the infant. He also described the range of components, implications, and conditions for initiating and maintaining this infant-mother bond in his work on attachment. Bowlby further noted that it is the quality of this bond that is the most crucial for developing and maintaining the psychological health and resilience of the individual throughout life. This concept is also extensively echoed in the work of Hilde Bruch who noted in 1941 that the conditions facilitating the development of obesity in children relate to a disturbance in this primal bond and a consequent lack of nurture.

Skubal (2002) proceeds from the ego-identity and presents the oral in the context of cultural identity and assimilation in eating. She defines disordered eating simply: as eating too much or too little, or to mean idiosyncratic eating habits such as restricting oneself to one food group only. She also noted that the entire range of classification of eating disorders rests on a simple premise: that eating, like other culturally controlled acts, needs to be ordered. Skubal is quick to point out that the range of order is subject to changes in culture—what we define as binge eating and *bulimia* today was in fact the very epitome of cultured and polite society in ancient Rome, as told by Steward Lee Allen in his book *The Devil's Garden* (2003), when no civilised household would be found without a *vomitorium*—the place where guests would literally purge themselves after episodes of binge eating (a common feature of the Roman banquet), only to repeat the cycle again.

According to Skubal, the modern obsession with obesity arises from the ideal body weight norms promoted by insurance companies and this obsession with the ideal body presents as a type of hyper-order in that it seeks control of appetite, weight, and ultimately the body itself. However, as can be seen in the work of Caroline Bynum of 1987, disordered eating is not new, with poets and historians of the ancient past noting cases of refusal to eat as aberrant, and gluttony as the first of the seven deadly sins (Skubal, 2002) long before eating disorders became the subject of medical and sociological inquiry. Nonetheless,

Skubal cautions that in this context of cultural change, when writing about eating disorders, one must distinguish between the prevailing "cultural cult of thinness—the anorexic ideal" as Paul Campos terms it in 2004. Skubal noted that in terms of pounds and inches, given this anorexic ideal, it is harder now than at any other time in history to be considering eating disorders on the anorexic side of the scale, although the reverse may well be true on the "overweight" or obesity side of the spectrum. Given the almost universal drive to leanness that dominates popular culture, the ordered dieting, even fasting girl "merely impersonates the pathological" (Skubal, 2002, p. 69). She noted that several studies have similarities in the origins of both obesity and its opposite, *anorexia nervosa*. For example, women, in particular, are more likely to succumb to eating disorders due to their proximity to food production, preparation, and consumption which trace in turn the effects of a patriarchal and objectifying culture that has "shaped and shocked and shamed the female body into girdles and fat farms and frailty" (p. 70). These concepts are explored further in Chapter Five.

The unconscious and neuroscience

Insofar as the contribution of the psychoanalytic approach to the treatment of obesity is concerned, Bruch noted some limitations in that the approach is built on the theory of drives, particularly as far as Freud is concerned and while "psychoanalytic concepts helped to clarify the psychodynamics of disturbed eating behaviour and the symbolic significance of food and body size, they were not effective in therapeutic applications" (Bruch, 1961, p. 53).

Despite these misgivings, the idea of the unconscious has found support in neuroscience which has confirmed the existence of unconscious mental processing, according to Elizabeth Phelps and Joseph Le Doux (2005), and unconscious memory processing following brain injury, according to Richard Bryant (2001). Similarly, Phelps and Le Doux found that irrational fear responses and other abnormal behavioural patterns are based in the bypassing of the hippocampus, which contains conscious memory. As the hippocampus is bypassed, the conscious cortex is connected to the primitive brain structures thus triggering unconscious memories of early trauma, thereby supporting Freud's contention that neuroses originate in the traumas of childhood.

The unconscious, neuroscience, and obesity

Applied to the problem of obesity, John Gunstad and associates (2006) showed that the tendency towards obesity originates in the early maladaptive programming of the brain, linking to Freud's theory that the *id* is not ruled by the reality principle, but rather the pleasure principle, and that this is the factor that renders rational and conscious decisions to make the lifestyle changes necessary to combat obesity ineffective over the long run, for the simple reason that obesity is not seen as a problem by the *id* which is ruled by the pleasure principle. It is this particular instinctual and unconscious pleasure-seeking behaviour of the *id*, further supported by the endogenous neurological pathways for addiction including the endocannabinoid system, according to Tim Kirkham and Sonia Tucci (2006), that conspires to completely overrule the conscious efforts of those seeking to overcome obesity to implement the necessary lifestyle changes consistently. It continues to provoke the wishful thinking, denial, and illusions that so often present in people with obesity as they seek to rationalise their behaviour. While psychoactive medication presents much promise in the treatment of obesity, the moderation of the neurochemical pleasure-seeking systems must be combined with a therapeutic intervention that draws from the lessons of psychoanalysis as these may help in unearthing early trauma, complexes, fears, anxiety, and unconscious conflicts which determine the specific pathways to seeking pleasure and sustain the pathology underlying obesity.

The research that is available shows that there is a vast number of factors that need to be considered when looking at obesity and addressing the coalescing eating behaviour. The theories of obesity discussed in Chapter Two offered different methods that could be implemented to improve lifestyle and reduce obesity, but many if not all of these programmes have to be used in conjunction with other programmes to gain results.

The psychoanalytic theory: Jung

The theory of the transcendent function

Jung believed that conflict arises when two opposite tensions have equally strong motives. The ego and the unconscious are a battle between two forces, both refusing to surrender. The result of the stagnant situation is the rise of a third force that Jung called the transcendent function. Transcendent function is a tension between the conscious and the unconscious that works towards unification through exploration and integration of new directions to produce a whole new insight, resulting in a deeper sense of self, as explained by J. C. Miller (2004).

Jung's transcendent function results through the purposive unconscious. Jung believed that the ultimate achievement of human self-realisation, which he called *individuation*, could only happen through the transcendent function (Jung, 1969, p. 275). Miller explains that Jung marked the activation of the transcendent function as a sign of progression towards maturity and the unity of the self.

Jung believed that symbols were created by the "fantasy-producing activity of the psyche" (Jung, 1969, p. 4) and that it served as a bridge between the conscious and unconscious in order to achieve integration and new direction. The symbol for Jung was not a compromise that was reached between the conscious and the unconscious, or a combination of ideas that has been integrated, but rather a new perspective, or as Jung explains it, a "living, third thing ... a living birth that leads to a new level of being, a new situation" (1960, p. 90), and as such the symbol is the facilitator that reconciles psychological opposites.

These symbols seep through to the conscious through dreams, and by recognising these symbols and learning to understand the significance of them in our lives, we achieve differentiation and detachment by treating our thoughts as objects and separating them from the emotion that is triggering the thought. The detachment allows for the reconciliation of opposites and, if not achieved, Jung warned that the self was at risk of dissolution into counter partial sets, as Dr. A.J. Drenth explained in 2016. To remove the tension arising from the two opposing forces, Jung advocated the separation of awareness itself from the contents of awareness. The libido, for example, is a form of tension or energy that could be removed to ease the process emerging into the unconsciousness to explore the symbols, images, and fantasies that seep through to the conscious. The symbol thus serves as a common channel through which the two opposing forces can flow in order to find common ground to create a new alternative.

Jung proposed active imagination to activate the psyche "through an image or a chain of images and their related associations" (Schaverien, 2005, p.128) to bring unconscious thoughts or issues to the conscious. According to Joy Schaverien in his writings of 2005, the activation can only take place if there is a psychological split where the one part of the personality surrenders to and explores the fantasy (irrationality) and experiences the fantasy of the waking dream, while the other part of the personality observes the process (rationality). Jung explains that active imagination evokes archetypical material and relates to the collective unconscious.

Schaverien suggests methods to generate active imagination, which include creative expression such as dance movement therapy, sand play, and music to initiate the process of active imagination revealed as visualised imagery in both waking and sleeping dreams. In turn, it enables the understanding of both the patient's will to change and their resistance to change. The waking dream differs from a sleeping dream in that the consciousness is lowered intentionally to allow images to seep through to the consciousness. These events or images then appear in the consciousness as if it is reality. Schaverien describes this form of active imagination as a "lived experience" in which "the image generates psychological movement whilst the ego is held in a suspended state" (2005, p. 131).

Gaston Bachelard explains in 1964 that the concept of active imagination is an integral part of psychoanalysis, because it sets the client in motion, to move from the familiar to the unfamiliar and allows the client to embark on the exploratory road of fantasy by breaking the chains of the self and reality. The initial activation of active imagination is triggered by the therapist and used as a lens to explore the actual and illusory characteristics of the client, as well as certain patterns that manifest and feature in the patient's life. The therapist in turn can recognise presenting archetypal information and also interpret and analyse the relevance of the hidden mythology attached to the client's experience or imagery to help with the process of transference and understanding of the client's complexes.

Complexes and the treatment thereof could be a very traumatic experience. Often, after the complex or traumatic event has been processed, the initial memory of such an event may still be quite painful emotionally or distressing. The memory or trigger of the event of original traumatic experience will depend mostly on three factors. First, the degree of personal trauma that the person has experienced during the original event; second, the time that has elapsed since the processing and transcendent function of the event, and third, if the transcendent function has been done sufficiently.

When the event has been sufficiently processed through using transcendent exercises, the trauma will be triggered and can still result in initial trauma. The mind should immediately switch over to the transcendent function of the memory to alleviate discomfort. In some cases, it might be possible that the mind immediately switches over to the transcendent function memory (especially as time lapses), but in other instances the person has to consciously think of the transcendent memory in order to alleviate the emotional memories.

Here is an example to explain the concept. One bright and sunny day, a woman was walking with her small, fluffy dog on a big open patch of greenery. The woman and the dog had been companions for the last twelve years and did everything together, including daily walks in the neighbourhood or along the beach. The woman was always very diligent with putting her dog on a leash whenever there were other people or dogs in close vicinity, not because her dog was aggressive or uncontrollable, but rather to be able to protect him should other dogs become aggressive. As they were walking on the big open green space, no one was about and she let her dog run around without his leash. She did not notice that somebody had arrived from work behind her and opened the gate to drive his car into his yard. The man did not see her and she did not see the man. The next moment, the man's bull terrier stormed out of the gate, grabbed the small fluffy dog and shook him like a rag. The woman was screaming at the bull terrier to let him go. She saw her dog's terrified eyes and she thought that the bull terrier was going to kill her dog at that moment. She pushed her hand into the bull terrier's mouth, trying to ease his grip on her dog. By that time the owner was also there and attempted to tear the bull terrier away from her dog. After some excruciating minutes, and after biting both the woman and his owner, the terrier let go of her dog. Needless to say, the woman and her dog were both severely traumatised, bloody and sore, but lived to tell the tale.

The result of this frightening event was that the woman never took her dog for a walk for several months thereafter, hindered by the memory of that traumatic day and fear of its repetition.

After about eight months, one day a friend told her that she walks with a taser in her hand when she takes her four small dogs for a walk along the beach. When aggressive dogs come close, she presses the button on the taser, which makes a load sound, usually causing the aggressive dogs to retreat immediately. The woman took about another month to pluck up the courage to go for a walk with her dog again. She was armed with her taser and although it was very stressful for the both of them, they enjoyed being out and about again. From there they resumed their daily walks.

Regardless of the fact that life went on as normal, the trauma of that day was stored in the unconscious. Many different triggers would take the woman right back to that moment. The sight of any bull terrier, even on television; a charging dog no matter the shape or size; random memory flashes of that event and loving moments between the woman and her dog reminded her that she almost lost her fluffy companion.

Later, in initiating the transcendent function, the woman was guided to form three images in her mind:

Image one: She had to think about their walks and how life had always been before the attack.

Image two: She had to think about the attack itself and remember the emotions of that time.

Image three: She had to think of an alternative: what could have been done in order to alleviate the trauma of this event? In this case, the woman pictured that she had her taser in her hand and as soon as she saw the bull terrier attacking her dog, she pressed the button to make the noise. If that did not work, she would taser the bull terrier directly to incapacitate him and let go of her dog. Now every time the memory is triggered, instead of remembering the traumatic emotions, the woman will consciously remember the transcendent image and she will feel less helpless and emotional about the event.

In studying the above example, it is simple to recognise the challenges with processing a traumatic event successfully through the transcendent function. One of the most significant challenges with transcendent exercises is that the original trauma has to be remembered. The original trauma and its attached emotions that lay dormant in the unconscious have to be made conscious in order to sufficiently process and resolve the trauma. The person will have to connect the current triggered emotions with the original traumatic event, so that when the unconscious triggers the specific emotion, the person will consciously recognise the complex or the original trauma. In order to alleviate the attached traumatic emotions, the person will thus recall the new transcendent image.

It is important to note that the trauma does not simply disappear after the transcendent function has taken place; the trauma will always remain. Instead of triggers of the event that result in uncontrollable emotions and turmoil, she will still remember what happened, but now she also remembers the transcendent image and this alleviates the painful emotions that were experienced that day. In other words, the person is in charge of how she reacts to the trigger. So now, every time a trigger to the event is presented in her life, instead of experiencing the same traumatic emotions that she did at the event, she now can consciously acknowledge the trigger and process it through the new transcendent image to alleviate the pain of reliving that moment.

The above is a simplified example in that the complexes and triggers were easily identified as she was aware of the traumatic event that took place. The process of the transcendent function becomes much more complicated when the trauma occurred during childhood, for example, and has been dormant in the unconscious for many years. It is important to remember that when trauma is stored in the unconscious, it is because the trauma is too unbearable for that person to deal with the emotions at that time on a conscious level, and in order to proceed as normal with daily events, the mind's automatic response is to store those events in the unconscious. Triggers of the event then unsettle the unconscious and cause unexplainable emotions. This is what is called our complexes.

THUS:

Complexes = a traumatic event (stored in the unconscious) + irrational emotions (experienced in the conscious).

The next important factor to take note of is that complexes are not necessarily the result of an event that was traumatic. It can also be a good or positive event that took place and triggers negative emotions later in life.

Here is an example to explain the phenomenon:

A young, obese woman in her late thirties was doing a course on symbols with a Jungian institution and students were asked to identify significant symbols in their everyday lives. When she received the first module material on the Friday, the seed was planted, her mind was immediately activated to recognise her own symbols.

She struggled to recognise her symbols, and then it happened … Since the weekend before, there was a piece of chocolate cake sitting under the glass cake dome in her kitchen. As she decided on Monday (like every Monday) to start on a diet, she consciously coaxed herself to not allow the cake to bother her and to allow someone else to finish it.

Every time she went to the kitchen, she was aware of the chocolate cake on the worktop. On the Wednesday her partner ate a piece of the chocolate cake when she came home from work. It did not bother her and she was not in the least tempted to have a piece. On Thursday the same thing happened. Still there was no problem.

The problem came on Friday. After working in her study at home the whole morning, she walked into the kitchen to make some tea (please note that the cake is now seven days old). She could not resist it any longer. She HAD to have it. Her whole being was depending on that piece of chocolate cake. Her sanity was hanging on a thread for that piece of chocolate cake. She opened the dome. She ate it. It was dry and it was too sweet, but oh boy was it good, she thought. From there the binging started … a piece of chocolate … a piece of bread … etc. Needless to say, that was the end of her diet for the weekend.

She knew that the piece of left-over chocolate was symbolising something, but she just could not figure it out or perhaps did not want to acknowledge it. For five days she was contemplating it in the back of her mind, but she just could not put her finger on it.

The Tuesday night, in the middle of the night while thinking of Jung, the course, and the exercise, she thought again of the mystery of the left-over chocolate cake and decided to take it step by step.

She asked what chocolate cake reminded her of.

It reminded her of times when she was small and her mother used to bake a chocolate cake for special occasions, either when people were coming to visit or somebody in the family's birthday. As a child, she was allowed to help with the mixing of the cake ingredients and her mother allowed her to lick out the bowl of icing when she was done decorating the cake. The chocolate reminded her of the special moments in her childhood days. Some evenings, after watching the news on television, she would go with her father to the shop to buy bread. He always bought sweets which they would eat while driving home. It was "their little thing" and usually it was the highlight of her day. She started to understand the emotion. The cake never bothered her until she was alone. The chocolate cake and the chocolate symbolised that "togetherness" and that feeling of love and nurture. That is why when she ate that piece of chocolate cake, it didn't even taste good physically, but it satisfied her mentally. Her mental hunger for love and nurture was fulfilled.

This only raised more confusion for her. She had always perceived herself as a loner and feeling comfortable with being alone. Where was this emotion coming from? When she was creative, writing, or busy with something that she enjoys she was fine. But during the day, when she felt lonely, she would seek "comfort" ... food.

Unfortunately, or perhaps fortunately with the application of transcendent exercises, if one can of worms is opened, a domino effect takes place and by thus raising one complex, many other complexes or related issues might arise that need pondering. In the above case: why was she scared to be alone during the day? The question brought up a few events that happened when she was a child and two incidents when she was alone at home as a child.

In order to resolve the current emotion that was causing dysfunction in her life, she could now recall those two events, and apply the transcendent function exercise in order to deal with the emotion of those events to solve the current "almost unexplainable" emotions. The bridge between the trauma stored during her childhood, in the unconscious, and the unexplainable emotions currently experienced consciously, could now be built to change the symbolism attached to the complex, in order to understand the current experienced emotion and also to be able to react differently when triggers arise through transcendence. Thus, she decided, transcendent exercises should be applied if she wishes not to seek love and nurture in food every time she is alone.

However, one should never forget that "change is difficult" as the famous author Victor Frankl (1984) observed. The trauma has been stored in the unconscious for the person to proceed with daily duties as per normal. Recalling the stored trauma can be very disturbing, therefore in many instances these traumas have been stored so deep in the unconscious that a person might not remember them at all, and often the person is not even aware of the existence of these traumas that have lain dormant in the unconscious. These complexes can only be recalled when the psyche feels that the person is ready to deal with the trauma or old/wise enough to wish to do so. This is a very important note: "if the person should wish to". The person might start to remember flashes of the event and at this stage can choose to engage with the symbol that is presented by the unconscious or not. It is important to never force a person to deal with these complexes as each person is on his or her own life's journey and there is no right or wrong method to deal with complexes. When the time is right or when she feels she is ready for the next part of her developmental journey, she can engage with her unconscious. Now that she has learned that she is uncomfortable with being alone at home and seeks comfort in food to alleviate that unexplainable emotion, she is aware that there is "something". The unconscious has been triggered. She may begin to receive flashes or what can also be called symbols from the unconscious. She might start thinking about the flash that she just had. "What was that?" And the more she will think about the flashback, the more the memory takes shape around that flashback. Now instead of only remembering the one single picture of the event, she begins to experience the event as she did at the time and she remembers the emotions that she felt during that time. With the transcendent function it is important to connect the emotion felt during this exercise with the similar emotions that she is experiencing as an adult. Perhaps it is shame, anger, sadness … whatever emotion she felt during that traumatic event will surface later in adult life if unprocessed.

Jung called these suppressed events in the unconscious, complexes. With good reason: it is a very complex subject indeed. The psyche suppresses these events in the unconscious, because it is dealing with events that we do not want to face voluntarily. It is heavy and difficult to face and painful to remember. We should never underestimate the immense influence of these complexes on our everyday lives. There are things we do automatically and without thinking twice about it, but essentially the complexes remain deeply rooted in the unconscious.

Jung's perceptions of the conscious and unconscious

The similarities between Freud and Jung are found in their agreement that the human psyche consists of separate, but interacting systems, the main ones being the ego, the personal unconscious, and the collective unconscious, and like Freud, Jung also emphasised the importance of the personal unconscious in the development of personality. Jung diverged from using Freud's concepts of the id, the ego, and the super-ego and also distanced himself from Freud's sexual theory. Jung felt that the deep unconscious forces were revealed through mysticism, dreams, and religious beliefs as the means of conscious expression.

To Jung, the ego represented the *conscious mind* including the thoughts, memories, and emotional content the individual is aware of, and as such, the ego enables identity and continuity. The *unconscious* for Jung consisted of two layers; the first, the *personal unconscious* is essentially similar to Freud's concept of the unconscious which describes it as consisting of temporarily forgotten information and repressed memories, but Jung added the concept of *complexes* to the personal unconscious. Jung saw complexes as a collection of thoughts, emotions, and memories focused on a single concept, and proposed that the more elements are attached to the complex, the greater its influence on the individual. Jung further argued that the personal unconscious was much nearer to the surface (conscious) than Freud suggested.

The concept of Jung's complexes explained

Daryl Sharp illustrated in 2001 the concept of complexes using the analogy of a boarding house in which different personalities cohabit, but generally do not interact much—until confrontation arises between them. As the peace and harmony in the boarding house is disturbed, the dynamics between the boarders manifest. Sharp describes complexes as "the building blocks of the psyche" (2001, p. 9) but sees them as neither negative nor positive forces, but merely existing. Yet, as these complexes activate our emotional responses to any given situation, they have a powerful impact on our lives. The triggered complex causes us to impulsively react out of the ordinary and consequently cloud our rational judgment. The power of complexes can become so intense that they can manifest as physical symptoms, such as heart palpitations, digestive disorders, or respiratory problems.

Sharp explains that as complexes are engrained in our existence, separation from them is impossible, and consequently they need to be recognised and understood to better control their impact on the human psyche. Jung's complexes echo Freud's theory of memories stored as symbols in the unconscious that trigger responses or reactions in the conscious.

While both Freud and Jung agreed that a person's behaviour is determined largely by past and childhood experiences, Jung included future aspirations as a determinant of behaviour. Jung also posited that the personal unconscious is much nearer to the surface than Freud suggested and consequently Jungian therapy is less concerned with repressed childhood memories, and more focused on the present and future, which Jung believed to be the key to both the analysis of neurosis and its subsequent treatment.

The collective unconscious and archetypes

The most marked difference between Jung's unconscious and the version put forward by Freud was Jung's addition of the concept of *the collective unconscious* or transpersonal unconscious which he described as the level of consciousness shared with other people as it comprised latent memories of our ancestral and evolutionary past. He argued that "the form of the world into which [a person] is born is already inborn in him, as a virtual image" (Jung, 1953, p. 188), and the human mind has innate characteristics, such as the fear of spiders or the dark, as a result of our early evolution. This insight led to Jung's development of the archetypes as he argued that some aspects of the collective unconscious developed into separate subsystems of the human personality. Consequently, these ancestral memories and images (the archetypes) have universal meanings across cultures, and evidence of their existence tends to show up in very similar symbols in dreams, literature, art, and religion across the world.

Given this basis, Jung concluded that humanity's primitive past—as contained by the archetypes—forms the basis of the human psyche, which influences and directs human behaviour. Jung identified several archetypes including the *persona* (or *mask*) as the outward face of conformity we present to the world, but which also conceals those aspects of our real self which are non-conforming and thus not presented publicly.

The concept of the anima and animus explained

Jung described the anima as the female energy present in all of us; in men, the anima is the "syzygy" which is a man's instinctual and sensitive side, or put differently, his sixth sense of perception. The power of the anima in a man presents in his mood and gut feeling, and the energy in which the anima influences the man's life is largely a function of his relationship with his mother. A negative or complex and troublesome mother-son relationship tends to lead to a negative anima in the son (which in Freudian terms would play out as the Eros/Thanatos archetype) which he would experience as a negative energy translating into an oversensitive and defensive nature, petulance, apprehension, and in some cases, depression. For the male energy of the animus to be strengthened in men, they have to overcome the challenges of the negative anima, for if not dealt with, the anima can be incredibly destructive and in some instances the source of severe depression leading to suicide.

Archetype: anima and animus

The *anima/animus* as the mirror image of the biological gender is the unconscious femininity in males and the unconscious masculinity in females, and developed as a result of men and women cohabiting for millennia. Jung particularly focused on the *anima/animus* arguing that as men were discouraged from expressing their feminine tendencies and women their masculine tendencies, the development of both male and female in Western society was fundamentally undermined. Going further, Jung proposed that the patriarchal nature of Western society devalued the feminine qualities altogether and that in an overly conformist world, the predominance of the persona/mask has elevated insincerity to become an unquestioned way of life as people became even more alienated from their instinctual selves.

Jung's theory of the archetypical anima and animus applied to obesity

Applied to obesity, Marion Goodman noted in 1980 that women in reaction to a male-dominated society and culture sought to fit in by adopting male characteristics including competitiveness and goal-oriented behaviour, thus emphasising the masculine *animus*, and failing to feed their unconscious feminine principle, the *anima*. When the forces of the anima and animus are no longer in balance, pathology follows, and in the case of women, the unconscious femininity manifests in somatic form either as the devourer of the anorexic or as the obese using the image of the Great Goddess. Goodman contends that only by loving the goddess lost within her own rejected body can a woman hear her authentic voice and deal with the symptoms of anorexia and obesity.

Archetype: the shadow

The *shadow* is Jung's iteration of Freud's concept of the *id* in that it represents the animal spirits driving both the creative and destructive energies in the human psyche while the *self* provides the individual with a sense of unity in experience. For Jung, the ultimate aim of development was the achievement of a state of selfhood, and he argued that many of the societal problems he saw arising from the Cold War era as deriving from "man's progressive alienation from his instinctual foundation" (Jung, 2012, p. 44).

The relationship between archetypes and complexes explained

To connect the concept of archetypes with complexes, Daryl Sharp explained in 2001 that an archetype is at the core of any personal complex. For instance, the archetype of the mother can either symbolise nurturing or security or the archetype of the mother can be expressed as possessiveness or negligence. With Jung's discovery of the archetypes, he nullified the theory of people being "born into the world *tabula rasa*, a blank slate waiting to be writ upon by life" (Sharp, 2001, p. 13). As complexes, archetypes cannot manifest as a being or a definite object, but through mythology and many mythical tales, and they have been described and presented as creating a force with many different faces. Sharp defines an archetype as a "primordial, structural element of the human psyche" (2001, p. 14). Behaviour is a universal phenomenon; the creation of ideas and images is also a universal phenomenon. Instincts are the physical equivalents of archetypes and complexes are the personal reaction to an archetypal image. Sharp advocates it is the personal responsibility of each person to become aware of their complexes and manifestations in everyday life.

When conflict arises, there is a distortion between the conscious and the unconscious. More often than not, a rising conflict is not from an external cause, but rather from a trigger that activates a complex in the unconscious. Conflict that arises is thus often not caused by external triggers but rather unconscious triggers that can manifest as projection onto the person towards whom the conflicting emotions are directed. In other words, a person dislikes a certain personality trait, characteristic, or behaviour of another person; it is merely a reaction to one of someone's personal complexes of the unconscious which is causing a response in the conscious. Freud believed that these responses could best be dealt with if they are activated in the therapeutic session. This also coincides with Jung's theory, in that he believes that complexes cannot be brought to the conscious intentionally and can thus only be recognised in a conflict situation. Sharp brands conflict as the "hallmark of neurosis" (2001, p. 38). He describes it as conflicting poles of obligations and desires, and yet some conflict can be good, in order to self-explore and to self-realise and can act as a force for change. However, conflict becomes neurotic when it overtakes other facets of one's life or physically and mentally overwhelms the person.

Richard Evans depicted (Evans, Jung, & Jones, 1964) that the idea of archetypes was not well received by the Freudian camp, with Freud's biographer Ernest Jones noting that Jung "descended into a pseudo-philosophy out of which he never emerged", but the recurrence of mythological symbols in both contemporary culture and personal therapy suggests that Jung's archetypes may indeed reflect an innate cultural residue and ideas that once had survival value in the evolutionary context. Jung's work presented important ideas to the development of personality theory in that he was the first to distinguish the two main orientations of personality (introverted and extroverted) and also identified the four basic functions (thinking, feeling, sensing, and intuiting) which, in a cross classification, presented the eight major personality types subsequently developed further by Raymond Cattell's (1963) sixteen factor personality theory, Eysenck (Parish, 1965), and the Myers-Briggs Type Indicator (Kaplan & Saccuzzo, 2009).

The public break between the two followed, according to William McGuire's 1995 study of the letters between Jung and Freud, over Jung's public criticism of Freud's theory on the Oedipus complex and his emphasis on infantile sexuality. Freud proposed that the main motivational force from which both human behaviour and pathology derived was repressed and expressed through sexuality, which Freud explained in his theories on psychosexual development, notably as the *Oedipus* and *Electra* complexes. In the case of male children, Freud proposed that they have strong sexual desires for their mothers and resent their fathers; it is also during this developmental stage that the male children develop castration anxiety—the fear that their fathers will remove their penises as punishment for desiring the mother. The converse, the Electra complex, develops somewhat differently. It starts out with penis envy as the female child desires to have sexual relations with the mother, but realises she cannot do so in the absence of the penis. Consequently, she envies and desires the father's penis, which then progresses towards a sexual desire for the father and a resentment of the mother. Freud argued that these hidden desires would be repressed, but anxiety and defence mechanisms would later testify to their continued presence in the form of neurosis.

Freud's and Jung's perceptions of dreams

To Freud, dreams were the link to the unconscious; but to Jung, it was rather the phenomenon of the complexes that initiated not only dreams, but also symptoms, according to Daryl Sharp. Gaston Bachelard explained in his writings of 1964 that dreams are not a form of active imagination per se, but rather act as a converter to activate the imagination. Freud regarded dreams as a "wish-fulfilling and sleep-preserving function" (Sharp, 2001, p. 76). Freud distinguished between two kinds of dreams, the complex dream which entailed metaphorical images which was revealed through symbols. This type of dream coincided with Jung's understanding of the dream with "great vision, big, meaningful and of collective importance" which he regarded as extremely symbolic (Jung, 1928, p. 4). The other type of dream was named by Freud as the simple dream that might consist of events that happened during the day and do not carry many symbols. It is thus merely residue of a specific event that took place during the day. The simple dream also coincides with Jung's "ordinary small dream" and can be explained as the shallow dream with little or no symbolism. Jung regarded dreams as self-regulatory signs from the unconscious that act independently and spontaneously. Dreams are thus simply live commentary from the unconscious to digest life events. For Jung, the main purpose of dreams was to "compensate conscious attitudes—to call attention to different points of view—in order to produce an adjustment in the ego-personality" (Sharp, 2001, p. 76). Sharp describes the process of compensation as a harmonising measure between the forces of the unconscious and the conscious, in order to reach accord and win support from the conscious.

According to Jung, the solution to conflict that the client might be experiencing in his or her life might be revealed through symbols in the client's dreams. Thus, the dream reveals information to the consciousness in order to restore equilibrium in the psyche.

Unlike Freud, Jung did not attempt to determine the concealed meaning of dreams; he treated dreams as the "facts of the psyche" and rather attempted to associate the dreams with archetypes and personal context (Jung, 1934, p. 404). Joy Schaverien warned in 2005 that not every dream can be interpreted as active imagination that has seeped through from the unconscious. Material can arise from the unconscious, but it is up to the patient to be willing to investigate or explore the symbols that arise. If the client simply prefers to ignore or dismiss the arisen material, it returns to the unconscious and remains in hibernation. Even in the therapeutic setting, the therapist might show interest in a certain dream, but the client might be unwilling to explore the dream. Without the client's willingness to relate to the dream, transference is impossible. When the client refuses to acknowledge the symbols that have appeared from the unconscious, leaving them to hibernate; the unconscious intensifies the dreams and the dreams become repetitive as if the unconscious wants the material to be acknowledged in the conscious. When dreams are then noted in the conscious, they become weaker and less frequent.

By looking at the psychoanalytic theories of Freud and Jung, it becomes evident that the complexes of the unconscious and the willingness of the conscious to change thus play a vital role in the success of any weight loss or change intervention. The symbolism and its rich array of information that is hidden in the unconscious will be explored in the following chapters to determine the path from the unconscious complexes to the transcendence of the conscious.

CHAPTER 3

Concept one: symbols

The following chapters will discuss the literature of the five concepts: the collective unconscious, food, obesity, the personal unconscious, and symbols, in order to discover what the linkage is between food symbols and dietary behaviour leading to obesity. These five concepts will be discussed in sequence, and examples in the form of tales, such as *Alice in Wonderland* and *Hansel and Gretel*, will be used to illustrate the application of the Freudian and Jungian theories to the concept of the symbology of food.

In seeking to explain the underlying contributors of pathological eating behaviours—specifically obesity, it is important to explore the cultural and historical narratives of food and the symbolic meaning ascribed to it, as these considerations present the context of the constructs that a person forms around food, body image, and eating behaviour.

The interpretation of the literature selection is presented through the lens of the classic psychoanalytic theory as originally proposed by Freud in *An Outline of Psychoanalysis* (1940a) and in 1953 expanded on by Jung's analytical psychology in which symbols are the language of the unconscious.

Consequently, the chapter explores both symbol and myth, for this is the language of the unconscious, and the sociocultural narratives surrounding it.

What emerges from the historical analysis is that for long the medical opinion of obesity hardly changed, though it has advanced greatly in modern times. From the ancient healers, such as Galen and Aristotle, who recognised obesity as a health risk; to the Victorian times with William Banting's letters on corpulence; to modern scientific research regarding the pathways through which obesity manifests in other life-threatening health conditions such as diabetes, hypertension, and reduced quality of life and life expectancy, as stated by the World Health Organization, medicine through the ages seems to have adopted a consensus on the health risks associated with obesity.

Luke and Monica Roman explained in 2010 that until now the social, cultural, and mythological narrative appears to be very much a product of human social and cultural evolution through the ages. In ancient times, when agriculture was in its infancy and humans had very little control over the elements of nature and limited understanding of the science of food production, their food sources were anything but secure. Consequently, the narrative was very much one where abundance in food equalled being favoured by the gods, and being well-fed and corpulent was a sign of divine blessing and material well-being. Food played a central role in myth, religion, and ritual; for one to prosper, the gods had to be appeased. Unsurprisingly the ancient gods, who, as divine beings, were not subject to the variability of nature and suffered no famine, were all obese. Retaining a state of obesity implied an absolute control over nature, far removed from the limitations faced by humanity. To commune with the gods, the language of food was spoken.

In contrast during medieval times, characterised by periodic famine, pestilence, and war, and not being able to control nature to the extent where reliable food production was possible, the emergence of Christianity, mainly in the form of Catholicism resulted. However, for the Church to retain power over kingdoms and humanity as a whole, a narrative where abundance of food was evidence of the favour of God was not entirely sustainable, given that medieval society was far from food secure. Hence, the introduction of the suffering Jesus, gluttony as a cardinal sin, and sacrifice and self-denial as signs of communion with divinity, that promised favoured status and godly favour. It is in this context that the holy anorexics find their place, along with the self-denial commonly practised by the holy men and women of the age, as told by Thomas Aquino and Timothy McDermott (1997).

With the dawn of the age of reason in the eighteenth century, where humanity discovered new worlds, gained colonies, trade routes and technological advances and greater food security; the excessive consumption of food came into vogue again. This time excessive consumption occurred in the context of a material world and became symbols of wealth, prosperity, and power where the plump wives of rich men were celebrated again.

In time there followed the post-industrial age, still a material world, but one in which absolute control and excessive food production has been attained. In this era of mass production, now the distinction between rich and poor had to be redefined. The mass-produced foods of the industrial world, laden with cheap sugar substitutes, starch, preservatives, and flavour enhancers became the common man's fare, with obesity as its mark. The rich, educated, and powerful shifted to "real" foods: more expensive, never preserved or frozen, always fresh, and less laden with trans-fats and sugar. Thus, the lean, muscular shaped bodies became the new status symbols which were associated with health, wealth, and privilege, according to Aleid Brouwer (2008).

Much as the figs, bananas, and grapes of antiquity were symbols of the divine in ancient mythology, the whole, fresh, and unprocessed foods of the rich combined with a highly regimented lifestyle of exercise and strict control of eating habits are strong symbols. It is contrasted to the pre-packed television dinners of the lower classes, uncontrolled eating, and a lack of disciplined exercise of the lower income groups. The medieval ascetics were more holy than the rest of society, while the kings and queens of the era ruled by divine right; they were the ones who enjoyed the ultimate favour bestowed by God and could eat the sweet foods of the time. So too are the modern adherents of healthy lifestyles blessed; they are better educated, have stronger characters, and are winners compared to the losers of the lower classes. Where obesity was once a sign of the favour of the gods, it has now become a social stain. For food symbolises social discourse, identity, and one's place in the world, according to Brouwer. In times gone by, food symbolises the blessings of the gods necessary for survival, while in a modern world it denotes a key aspect of material success.

While the apples of the ancient world promised immortality (Garden of Hesperides) and wisdom—the knowledge of good and evil (Garden of Eden), as described by Luke and Monica Roman, whole foods, super foods, special supplements, and gene editing today promise the everlasting fountain of youth and immortality. This narrative has not changed and mankind continuously desires overall improvement, consecrations, and complete well-being, for it displays the evolutionary advantage of some over others. At its heart is food as a conscious social, political, and economic discourse, while in the unconscious the symbolic discourse is equally lively, explained by Richard Klein (1996).

Lastly, Chapters Six and Seven will offer brief applications of both the Freudian and Jungian approaches to obesity, with Hilde Bruch in 1973 explaining obesity as a lack of nurture in the Freudian tradition, while Marion Woodman offers the Jungian analysis in 1980, in this case explaining obesity as an incomplete development of the female psyche. Similar examples of both approaches are briefly given with respect to their opposites: anorexia, which is applied to the holy anorexics in the Freudian case as an example of unresolved sexual tension; while the work of Marion Woodman and Marie-Louise Von Franz offers the Jungian approach as a search for perfection and the impossible ideal of complete control. As mentioned earlier, the chapter includes an example of how the symbols of food offer insight into the journey of transformation and individuation by offering an analysis of the tale of *Hansel and Gretel*. The story starts with the problem of famine in the land which leads to the abandonment of the children and their struggle for survival and growth, illustrating the psychodynamic perspectives of both Freud and Jung. Its starting point is to consider the impacts of recent advances in other fields, including quantum physics and bioelectronics on the validity of Jung's concept of the collective unconscious and the interconnectedness between the physical and mental worlds and the unconscious. The insights offered by quantum physics explain Jung's archetypes as wave forms existing in a quantum state of potentiality in the cosmic mind that can and do translate to matter in the empirical world. In particular, the impact of wave forms on the expression of cellular genetics provided by bioelectronics offers support to Woodman who argued that the difference in the number of fat cells between obese and normal weight patients derive from their psyche, in particular the unconscious, which she further illustrates by exploring the complexes through a word association test devised by Jung. The differences between the Freudian and Jungian approaches are further illustrated in more depth and an application to the problem of obesity is offered through a further exploration of the archetypes.

The Alice texts of Lewis Carroll are used to further illustrate the application of both Jungian and Freudian approaches. Given the nature of the Alice texts, the anima/animus is explored in the Jungian reading of the text against the metaphor of the Hero's Journey of transformation towards individuation. In this reading, Alice is analysed as a character in the Jungian tradition of reading the dream as an act employed by the psyche to compensate for an imbalance in the psyche, in this case in the anima as represented by the Death Mother archetype.

The Freudian reading of the text focuses the analysis on the author Lewis Carroll and sees the dream as expressing repressed trauma. In particular, the Eros/Thanatos complex is explored. In Carroll's case, according to the highly sexualised Freudian reading of the text, the Eros/Thanatos imbalance is translated in the occurrence of the *vagina dentata* as represented by Carroll's fear of the aggressive feminine represented by adult women and his ideation of little girls.

Concept one: symbols

What is a symbol?

In searching for the symbolic meaning underpinning the narratives about food in the cultural-historical context, the book considers several working definitions of symbols in psychological literature starting with Joseph Campbell who defined a symbol as an "energy evoking and directing agent" (2002, p. 153). Campbell later expanded on the definition by explaining that a symbol shows both sense and meaning and thus is a dual concept. A symbol functions on three levels simultaneously: in waking consciousness, in the spiritual realm of the dream, and in the domain of the absolutely unknowable or the unconscious. In the first two domains, a symbol has meaning, but in the domain of the unknowable, it can only be sensed.

As an example, Campbell noted that modern judges serve not only as a sociological purpose (that of keeping order), but also represent a working mythology. If their positions were just another role in society, judges would wear ordinary business suits, but instead they wear the magisterial black robe, which is the symbol that serves to ritualise and mythologise the power of the judge as a necessary condition for the law to hold a moral power, beyond the mere coercive power of the state.

Myths communicated through symbols in cultures

Moving from symbol to myth, Campbell noted that myths were designed as a harmonising mediator between mind and body, and serve to put the mind in accord with the body which in turn needs to adopt a way of life in accordance with the dictates of nature. The early myths, in particular, serve to enable the psyche to participate without a sense of guilt in the necessary acts of life, which in early society were all about eating and killing. "The hunt became a ritual of sacrifice, and the hunters in turn performed acts of atonement to the departed spirits of the animals". In doing so a "magical, wonderful accord" grew between the hunter and the hunted "as if they were locked in a mystical, time-less cycle of death, burial, and resurrection; their art—the paintings on cave walls—and oral tradition gave form to the impulse we now call religion" (Campbell & Moyers 1991, p. xvii).

The symbol: mediator between the mind and survival needs. The Asmat tribe as example

Lyall Watson (1995) provides a powerful illustration of Campbell's con-cept in his description of cannibalistic practices among the Asmat, a tribe numbering approximately 20,000 living in the delta area of Irian on the Casuarina Coast of Indonesian New Guinea, who regularly practise cannibalism as a means to sustain ecological balance in an environment characterised by a perpetual shortage of good quality protein, necessi-tating cannibalism. Upon coming of age, an Asmat requires a canoe and an owom—a special name belonging to the domain of the sacred and mystic. Prior to initiation, Asmat children are given a spirit name by the village seer, but once they have acquired their own personalities, they need a human name—the owom. Often, the problem is that the owom is usually a name that is already given to another Asmat in a neighbour-ing village and therefore cannot be given again; it must be taken.

The Asmat, as part of the initiation ritual then set up a man-hunt, and the end result is the killing and eating of a man from the neighbouring vil-lage. The young initiate who has to lead the hunt then inherits the victim's name (the owom) and also his responsibilities, including the care of his family. In this manner, the ecological balance is sustained by constraining competition for hunting and fishing resources, and population growth by keeping the number of sexually active males under control; and the body of the male eaten serves the much-needed protein for the people of the village to keep them healthy; yet the duty of care is embedded into the very identity: the human name of the initiate. Because the whole hunting and cannibalistic tradition is cloaked in cultural and religious practice, the symbol serves as the mediator between the minds of men and their survival needs to justify this act: the magical accord between the hunter and the hunted, according to Campbell. In this social, cultural, and ecological context, cannibalism is acceptable and practised in an ethical manner. In other contexts, where similar ecological constraints (protein shortage threatening survival) and cultural accommodation of the practice are not present, cannibalism is regarded as pathological.

Analogy between symbols in mythology and the collective unconscious

Jung spoke of these ideas as archetypes of the unconscious. Jung's archetypes of the unconscious were manifestations of the organs of the body and their powers and are biologically grounded and hence universal—the collective unconscious in which the personal unconscious finds its place. In contrast, Freud's unconscious is a highly personal unconscious as it is a collection of repressed traumatic experiences from the individual's lifetime, according to Campbell.

Campbell's definition of symbols not only focuses on the nature and persistence of symbols when he describes symbols as concepts and words, but also as visions, rituals, and images. Symbols for Campbell mirror reality; they hold the mind *to* truth but are not *themselves* truth. Miranda Bruce-Mitford (2008) sees a symbol as an image that represents an idea—the deeper indicator of a universal truth. As such symbols are the means for complex communication and often have multiple levels of meaning which is the characteristic that separates them from signs (only one meaning). Symbols are used to express and represent social structures and to represent specific aspects of culture and carry meanings that are culturally learned and not dependent on the symbol itself. Erving Goffman (1959) explained that symbols serve as the basis of human understanding of the world around us, and as the grounds for human judgment, as well as the basis on which humans identify with and cooperate within a community. Jung, von Franz, Henderson, Jacobi, and Jaffé (1964) proposed the initial distinction between sign and symbol described by Bruce-Mitford, in that signs stand for something that is known, while symbols represent the unknown and that which cannot be made clear or precise. To this he added the concept of archetype which is the larger concept of symbol, for example Christ would be the symbol of the archetype called *self*. The symbol's domain is thus the unconscious where it originates, and from where it is the impetus for conscious behaviour; including food pathology.

How symbols are formed

Food is part of everyday life and it becomes a very strong symbol for many facets of our lives. The symbolic power of food is enhanced by the evocation of all the senses and the extent to which it triggers an emotive response, which in turn depends on the mental associations that were created in the individual. These associations also determine how the food is perceived. Symbols can also develop rationally, spontaneously, over time, and through everyday usage, often called "organic symbols" as coined by Solomon Kats and William Weaver in 2013.

Victor Turner explains three anthropological properties of symbolism: condensation, which is used as an umbrella term for many ideas; unification, of symbols that link different orientations with each other, and polarisation of meaning. Given these properties of symbolism, the symbols attain their meaning through merging beliefs and feelings on the one end of the pole with an object on the other end of the pole. This results in a meaningful sensation or an experience that has meaning. For example, the American symbolism of the apple pie is explained by Kats and Weaver as a representation of not only the loyalty and cultivation Americans feel for their country, but it also represents the emotional strength and power that individuals feel to be part of this united nation. Interestingly, in the general parlance apple pie is also associated with motherhood. Kats and Weaver conclude that symbolism plays a prominent role in communication, not only between individuals, but also across generations.

The symbology of food as an element of the collective unconscious interacting with the personal unconscious

The symbology of food is proposed in this book as a working interaction of the symbols and archetypes of the collective unconscious with those of the personal unconscious. The symbols as they relate to food throughout history are presented, and core themes emerge in how they relate to the social order and the representation of the inherent power dynamic underpinning any social order. In keeping with the idea of an interconnected universe (the cosmic mind), it follows that the interaction of form and matter is multidirectional. As we draw archetypical images into our unconscious from the collective unconscious, so too do we draw forms from the environmental and social context within which we exist; which, if the logic is applied full circle, means that the social order and the power dynamics we see manifested there are in themselves manifestations of the collective consciousness of the time. In this sense the impact on the individual psyche of the social forces of the day cannot be ignored.

On the symbolism and value of dreams

Jung explained the symbolism in dreams as follows:

> Dreams are impartial, spontaneous products of the unconscious psyche, outside the control of the will. They are pure nature; they show us the unvarnished, natural truth, and are therefore fitted, as nothing else is, to give us back an attitude that accords with our basic human nature when our consciousness has strayed too far from its foundations and run into an impasse. (Jung, 1964, Collected Works, Volume 10, paragraph 317)

Jung saw the psyche as consisting of the mind, body, and emotions as all working together so that when imbalance occurs in the psyche, negative emotions or symptoms are helpful in drawing attention to it. As a self-regulating system, the psyche with all of its contents including dreams, thoughts, and feelings is what Jung termed "purposive". Consequently, the value of the dream as Jung saw it is as the psyche's attempt to communicate important contents of the unconscious to the individual. Dreams are also an important factor in the development of personality—a process termed by Jung as individuation.

This was in contrast to Freud, who posited that dreams are the expression of forbidden and suppressed wishes that have to be disguised in the form of a dream, distinguishing between the openly expressed surface content of the dream and the hidden latent content of it. For Jung, dreams expressed content openly. Jung wrote: "They do not deceive, they do not lie, they do not distort or disguise … They are invariably seeking to express something that the ego does not know and does not understand" (Jung, 1964, Collected Works, Volume 10 paragraph 189). Hence, Jung explained that if dreams appear to be difficult to comprehend, it is because their language of expression is symbol, and to understand the symbol is to understand the dream. He wrote that "A symbol is the best possible formulation of a relatively unknown psychic content," and that the dream is "a spontaneous self-portrayal, in symbolic form, of the actual situation in the unconscious" (Jung, 1964, Collected Works, Volume 10, paragraph 505).

To interpret dreams, Jung would identify the symbols in the dream and ask the patient regarding their associations with these symbols. "Only then does the meaning of the dream become apparent" (Jung, 1963, Collected Works, Volume 7, paragraph 123). However, the meanings of dreams occur both on the objective level—which would treat the dream images as corresponding to objects in the real world, and on the subjective level—these images or symbols correspond to elements in the individual's own psyche, which is where Jung focused his interpretation.

The amplification of dreams occurs when the personal dream symbol of the individual links with the broader, mythological meaning of the symbol—such amplifications could reference any kind of mythical, religious, fairy tale, or archetypical association. It is the amplification aspect of dreams which relates the dream to the archetypical level and accesses the content of the collective unconscious—that is, those aspects of the psyche which are universal to all of us, such as the animus, or masculine nature, for example.

However, when confronted consciously with the archetype, such as telling a woman she has a strong masculine nature, she might not agree as her conscious perception differs. Dream images correspond to the elements of the individual psyche, but they can also correspond to people in the real world, including the analyst insofar as the analyst may embody what the dream image is symbolising. It is in this context that transference between patient and analyst occurs. For this is the essence of the symbol, which can apply across different situations and to different people. By recognising the symbolic meaning of dream images as representation of the elements within the dreamer's own psyche, by identifying the dreamer's personal associations with the symbols, and then amplifying symbols in relation to archetypical themes, we are able to understand what the unconscious is communicating to the dreamer by means of the dream—usually by compensating for those aspects that are missing from or incomplete in the dreamer's conscious.

CHAPTER 4

Concept two: food

It all started with apples and tomatoes and ended up in polystyrene boxes ...

The nasty reality is that humanity's relationship with food has become corrupt on every level imaginable. We have obese people suffering from malnutrition due to lack of micronutrients in their diets, as stated in Damms-Machado, Weser, and Bischoff's article of 2012. Max Roser (2014) explains in his article that fertility levels are declining in the industrial world; and the impact of non-communicable diseases are directly attributable to poor diet and lifestyle choices, according to the World Health Organization (2003). They also express their concern that the lack of nutrition is fast becoming the main co-morbid association of communicable diseases, with poor sanitation and poverty of the early industrial and pre-industrial eras mentioned as the other dominating factors.

Despite all of our industrial and scientific advances, food security is on the decline as the environmental impacts of unsustainable production systems and the manner in which food is traded are coming home to roost. Giulia Soffiantini (2020) for example explained how the Arab Spring was in part a direct consequence of rapidly rising food prices due to the influence of commodity speculators on the food market. The industrial systems driving the production, distribution, and consumption of food are products of the age of reason, which brought us materialism and science. This overemphasis on the material world, which through the application of science became predictable and hence controllable, has solved many of the problems of the pre-industrial world. Food varieties were produced to be more drought resistant, farming practices were improved, and distribution systems developed to improve food hygiene and less spoilage. But in the search for higher volumes to keep feeding a growing global population (Markets and Markets, 2016), the large-scale industrial food production, distribution, and consumption system also made food impersonal, and took it out of its natural context of seasons and locality, and its connection with the divine.

Consider the cultural and religious practices of the pre-industrial world. Entire cultures developed around the foodstuffs that were available and gave raise to specific culinary traditions; to this day shallots form an essential part of the French cuisine, while the tortillas of the Mexican culinary tradition closely relate to the maize produced in the area. In contrast, when we think of rice, several traditions from the Japanese sticky rice essential to sushi to the long grain varieties of rice underpinning every Indian dish, and to the Indonesian rice table, pay tribute the different varieties of rice grown in the different regions of the world. Wheat underpins the baking traditions of Europe, and bread, whether made from wheat, sorghum, spelt, or maize is a perennial in every cultural tradition. The pre-industrial Church calendar still reflects the earlier times of festivals organised around food supply and its natural seasonal cycle. Practically every culture in the world has a harvest festival of sorts, of which the forty days fast of Lent can be used as an example. Lent is associated with sacrifice which incidentally reflects the time in the northern hemisphere when food is not so readily available after the winter period. Food also had a religious dimension; in the Judaeo-Christian tradition Jesus referred to himself as the "bread of life" and was born in Bethlehem (Beit-Lechem—literally translated as "the house of bread"). This dimension of food was universal.

Many mythical stories describe how tributes of food were brought to religious leaders and temples, and harvest festivals were held in places of worship, for before the age of reason, food was a gift from the gods, and the gods had to be kept happy and appeased at all times if natural disasters and poor harvests were to be averted and famine avoided. Food was also used for healing and the entire medical traditions of cultures across the world focused on food as healing, ranging from the Chinese, to the Mayans, and to the Druids. Today, with our ability to control the production of food independently of the gods, these cultural and religious traditions are left without anchor, and having extracted and mimicked the biochemical properties inherent in plants and other natural substances, our pharmaceutical industry is completely devoid of its original context. In pre-industrial society, the production of food had to be a co-operative effort; production was social, and so was consumption. The effects of disruption to the food system were local and collectively felt. In this world, food was nutrition; it was associated with religious and cultural concepts of nurturing and sustenance (Fouche, 2017). Post-industrial humanity, in which the body has become the machine, fuels the body as opposed to nurturing it; food has become fuel. It no longer is the end result; it is now an input into a productive system. Pre-industrial man worked so that he could eat. Post-industrial man eats so that he can work. The concept of "food" is changing in both meaning and substance. Food is no longer a cultural and religious construct; it is a commodity, and the human beings who consume it are consumers who consume individually and out of context. This change has had a profound impact, not only on our religious, social, and cultural systems, but also on our psyche; and for the most part, it is pathological, for a world which can landfill food in the face of starvation or which can modify food to the extent that it is disease giving is a world alienated from itself in very much the way Max Weber must have imagined. Weber introduced the concept of social alienation as a result of the rationalisation of production. In this he argued that people could no longer engage in any socially significant action unless they joined some form of organisation at the cost of their individuality (Elwell, 1996).

In this book, the basis of the pathology that food has become is explored. We can define it as pathology, on the basis that if the current trend persists, our food production, consumption, and distribution no longer serve to enhance the survival and vitality of the human species, but serve to undermine it. When the results of food consumption, distribution, and production deficiencies are threatening to become the leading cause of death in most parts of the world, then we are looking at food as a pathology.

What drives pathology in the psychological context is the unconscious, according to Jung, and the unconscious in turn is one without reason, acting purely on instinct and relates to our symbols. When these symbols become imbued with meaning in the unconscious and in turn drive conscious perception and behaviour, the process becomes an active *symbology*. If symbol is a construct, then *symbology* is a deconstructed version of the construct as a *process* very much in the manner in which the objective of learning is to form a construct, but the process of learning is to deconstruct. The pathology of our relationship with food manifests everywhere from the manner in which we produce food and how that leads to land grabs, the manner in which mass-produced food pursues profits at the cost of health, and how that is absolutely fine both morally and legally in most societies, to the commodification of food and the trading economics behind it, to how this food pathology impacts on the individual level. On one end of the spectrum are the "food as enemy" type anomalies which express in the form of anorexia nervosa and bulimia, to the food-as-additive substance, "food as emotional crutch" and "food as shame" spectrum of overweight to obesity. Woven in between are the physical aspects relating to the neurochemistry and the biochemistry of nutrition, to the sociology of body weight and the psychology behind it.

To explore the entire psychosocial universe of food would be impossible, and consequently the focus of this book is on a single problem: obesity. Yet, within obesity is an entire ecosystem of biology, neurology, psychosis, and sociology. Consider the case of some of the psychological causes of obesity; in one instance the pathology driving the behaviour is that of loss ("food as compensator" in harking back to an earlier time where food was associated with nurture and care), in another instance it is endocrinal dysfunction arising from a low-cost diet attributable to socialisation (limited food experience exposure) and socioeconomic circumstance.

Education in this instance could fail for another reason; low-income communities tend to share an external locus of control, so the relationship between cause and effect and the subsequent personal responsibility could be somewhat tenuous (J. Miller, 2005). There is the obesity-as-affluence in developing nations as tastes tend to move away from local produce to the "store-bought" phenomenon of fast food, and increased protein, fat, and sodium consumption. In other words: the dimension of food-as-addiction. No wonder there is little consensus in the weight loss world on what is the holy grail of weight loss; recent research, including Deniz Atalayer and his associates' (2013) that points to the hormonal precursor grehlin which, the logic goes, can be manipulated to control the appetite and therefore by deductive logic may lead to weight loss. Fine, if we are eating because we are hungry. Very many obese people don't and neither does the recently dumped student flattening two litres of ice cream in a fit of rage and sorrow (or the student who may prefer a stronger version of sugar—alcohol) but the reaction is the same.

These point to a neurological chain of events, which if repeated often enough becomes habit depending on personality, genetics, and a host of other factors. Food can also be a source of judgment: overweight people are often perceived as lazy and less capable, or suffering from lack of self-control, and Susan Averett's study (2019) showed that being overweight in the labour market often translates as a lesser likelihood of being hired in the first place, and should one be, one is likely to be hired at a lower salary. Entering the socioeconomic cycle again; many studies have shown that one is more likely to be overweight in an industrial country if one is poor—for processed food is cheaper, and one stays poor because one's job and remuneration prospects are limited by being overweight, and on top of that, one's time in the labour market is limited by the health impact of one's weight. It is a never-ending cycle.

The problem of obesity also presents on another level of complexity: it is not that we do not know what causes weight gain and how to lose it. We know more now than ever before. How then did generations before us not know the extreme levels of obesity and overweight that we are confronted with today? Sedentary lifestyles and processed foods, including a far higher prevalence of convenience foods, laden with unprecedented levels of sugar and fat, contribute to the problem, but still do not explain why the majority of the 7 billion people on the globe do not suffer from excess weight—although admittedly, if current trends persist, that may not be true in future.

The majority of weight loss programmes address the problem of excess weight with a simple equation; calories consumed must be less than calories burnt, and the resulting caloric deficit would lead to weight loss, hence the restrictive caloric eating programmes combined with exercise regimes. Enter Weight Watchers, and any other dietary regime that runs on caloric calculation and substitution. But then, not all calories are equal. Recent quasi-experiments suggest (e.g. *That Sugar*

Film, 2015) that one can reduce overall caloric consumption and still pick up weight, if those calories are simple carbohydrates and in particular, sugar.

Treatments including cognitive behavioural therapy, family therapy, drugs, dietary counselling are all attempts to address the problem in the field of excess weight and obesity, but as only 2 to 5% of people succeed in keeping the weight off, it is clear that there are still missing pieces in the puzzle. This can work; but, as the statistics show, the weight loss is seldom sustained.

At the core of the issue is our relationship with food: both biologically, hardwired through evolution as a survival issue and our cultures; and socially, as food becomes social discourse and relations. The very essence of our issue with food is embedded in our unconscious. Consider the average dating relationship. He still takes her out to dinner. The symbolism—I can provide for you and the type of dinner I can afford is an expression of the lifestyle you can expect. At some point, she will cook him something. The symbolism: I can make a home and provide a nurturing environment to raise offspring in. Not only has our behaviour and reaction been created through our cultural relationship with food, but also through our personal experiences that are deeply imbedded in the unconscious. Consider the following case and how it is expressed in many cultures. The original version: child, warriors, friends, family returns home. Let us thank the gods for their safe return by slaughtering an animal of sorts (sacrifice), and because this is a thanking of the gods ceremony, we will do it next to water or somewhere on a mountain top under a sacred tree. The modern version: child, friends, family, wage-earner come home. We go to the local supermarket, buy some meat and enjoy a barbeque, preferably next to the swimming pool, a river, or the sea, but a cluster of trees for shade on a summer afternoon will also do.

The mere fact that we seek "comfort food" when bored or disappointed shows that there is a story hidden deep within or an emotional connection. There may also be a biochemical basis for the choice of comfort food—interesting that the choice of comfort food always involves sugar and/or carbohydrates. By exploring the narratives that have been carried over through traditions relating to food, we might discover some of our core beliefs that have been woven into our behaviour towards food.

By exploring different cultures in the anthropological sense, periods in history and types of societies (agrarian, industrial, post-industrial) and the meaning they make of food, one can learn much about the unconscious dimension of food. Consider the food narrative of current post-industrial society (organic is good, caring, cultured, and sophisticated) with that of industrial society (store-bought food in excess was a mark of affluence and at a time when sugar was prohibitively expensive, pastries were the ultimate dainties), and that of agrarian society (where food was celebrated during harvest festivals), with the cultural narratives of taboos, and the message is clear; not only is food a cultural construct, it is a psychological construct too, embedded deep in the unconscious where it forms its own symbolism.

In this book we explore the *symbology* of food, meaning the interaction of human behaviour and symbols across history and also through cultures to discover the psychological impact that these symbols have on the unconscious of people. It is no accident that the most widely watched reality television programming is about food and the preparation thereof, also that cookbooks are still very popular in bookshops.

Jung and associates explained in 1964 that symbols are the communication channel between the conscious and the unconscious. Symbols are thus a representation of our core beliefs, the origin of our problems, and the reason for tendency towards self-destruction. Knowing one's symbols can possibly help to recognise one's patterns of self-destruction and consciously alter the way we make life decisions to improve our health or to live fuller lives. Jolande Jacobi described the phenomenon of symbols and interaction with the conscious as follows: "one can sometimes discover unexpected treasures in the unconscious, and by bringing them into consciousness strengthen his ego and give him the psychic energy he needs to grow into a mature person. That is the function of the powerful symbolism of our dreams" (Jung, von Franz, Henderson, Jacobi, & Jaffé, 1964, p. 274).

Maslow's theory of human behaviour (1943) presents a five-level hierarchy of needs with self-actualisation being on the fifth level, and the basic needs of food, shelter, and procreation being at the bottom. The hierarchy is progressive; one cannot really go to the next level unless the preceding levels of needs are met.

One might expect the present study to focus on the basic needs level (food for survival) but when food becomes a social and psychological construct, the distinction blurs. For example, if I master my sugar addiction and overcome decades of weight issues, I attain self-mastery which is a facet of self-actualisation, but if I do so to conform to the social body image, I am meeting a social need, lower on the hierarchy. The symbol drives the motivation, and it does so in unpredictable ways, as is the way of the unconscious. The first need is significant according to Werner Meyer, Cora Moore, and Henning Viljoen (2008), as the physiological requirements which involve the need to satisfy hunger or thirst, also to breathe and sleep, and for movement, sensations, and lastly sex are vital for the species' subsistence. Food is survival, and that survival need—like the others (safety and sex)—is a social quest, so food production becomes social, followed by food consumption—again social, but nowadays often very isolated.

Societies structure themselves around finding food, storing food, providing food for the ones that cannot yet provide for themselves, and ensuring future supplies of food. The form that structure takes tells us about the dominant values in that society. Where food becomes profit and health secondary, one lives in a predatory society in which the warrior and the charlatan are worshipped. The victim becomes the scapegoat for failing to mimic the dominant social theme. Consider the case of American politics. The indispensable nation quite openly celebrates the notion of American exceptionalism. The dominant theme in presidential debates is the ability of the United States to project geopolitical dominance. America cannot be anything but that shining city on the hill in this collective consciousness. It is also the most militarised, spied-on country in the world, engaged in perpetual warfare most of the time, and has some of the most predatory systems of banking and commerce known to mankind. It is also the most medicated, least healthy, and most obese society in the world; it has 48 m of its approximately 350 m population on food stamps, and one in five children goes to bed hungry. The overwhelming majority of the working class population in America are obese, but nutritionally deficient, and often have to choose between electricity for heating or eating or medicine (Pan, Sherry, Njai, & Blanck, 2012). The indispensable nation for all its geo-political dominance has a soft underbelly.

Evidently food has been the symbol of subsistence since the beginning of time. It is also the symbol of domination as we see. Symbolism is defined in the Oxford English Dictionary as "the use of symbols to represent ideas or qualities ... or style using symbolic images and indirect suggestion to express mystical ideas, emotions, and states of mind". Jung explains that a "word or an image is symbolic when it implies something more than its obvious and immediate meaning. It has a wider 'unconscious' aspect that is never precisely defined or fully explained" (Jung, von Franz, Henderson, Jacobi, & Jaffé, 1964, p. 4). Jung further explained that we use symbols to define phenomena that we cannot explain in words or are incapable of fully understanding. He used religion as a simple example to explain the concept of symbols. Each religion uses different symbols. The symbols associated with different religious groups have distinct meanings to their devotees, also to people outside these specific religions. In the case of food, consider the case of eggs: an almost universal symbol of fertility dating back to the time of Ishtar, which became Easter (funny how the bunny—rabbits are known for their prolific breeding—and the eggs persist). Yet, in isiXhosa culture, their consumption is forbidden to women of childbearing age. Similarly, Jung also explains that people can create their own symbols spontaneously through the dreams they have that can carry personal significance.

Personal rituals are often the result of assimilation of one's symbols; when we teach our children to share their sweets, it becomes habit and later becomes symbolic of caring for those around us. At the same time, conflict does not make for good dinner parties, and people fighting generally don't eat together, for the food tends to "stick in our throats". How and what types of food we share with others take on a meaning of their own. Very few white people in post-apartheid South Africa would think of serving the ubiquitous brown bread jam sandwich with very sweet tea or coffee to black people in a social context. Most of us consume bread, jam, sugar, tea, and coffee. But when one group serves that to another, it becomes a political symbol given our specific context. These personal symbols become part of everyday life and part of one's character and through regular, routine use become ritual, like the continued gifting of easter eggs that harks back to the fertility feast of Ishtar and that persists in the Christian celebration of Easter (D'Costa, 2013). The ritual, offering constancy, becomes a source of comfort and security, as explained by Amanda Harrist and associates in 2019.

The previous examples display how these rituals can become engrained in our character. It becomes automatic and soon we do not remember why the ritual was initiated, but the symbol of the ritual is forever engrained in the unconscious and handed down from generation to generation. Family and societal rituals are thus often enriched with symbols. Ember and Ember noted in 1988 that the phenomenon of integration into a specific society or culture is predominantly dependent on learning and understanding the culture's symbols.

Our "unconscious" which is our bank of symbols is described by Jung as follows:

> There are, moreover, unconscious aspects of our perception of reality. The first is the fact that even when our senses react to real phenomena, sights, and sounds, they are somehow translated from the realm of reality into that of the mind. Within the mind they become psychic events, whose ultimate nature is unknowable (for the psyche cannot know its own physical substance). Thus, every experience contains an indefinite number of unknown factors, not to speak of the fact that every concrete object is always unknown in certain respects, because we cannot know the ultimate nature of matter itself. (Jung, von Franz, Henderson, Jacobi, & Jaffé, 1964, pp. 4–5)

Freud described the unconscious level as part of the human psyche where the "forbidden" wishes and motivations, and their actual memories, are all stored. The emotions related to these thoughts or memories are thus not familiar to the conscious as it is stowed away in the unconscious. Meyer explains that the suppression of these thoughts, emotions and memories are thus a defence mechanism of the ego to protect itself from the real emotions and inner conflict that these events may produce (Meyer, Moore, & Viljoen, 2008).

The forbidden fruit in the Garden of Hesperides

"The apple's seductive colours, its two-faced flavour, its suggestively feminine core, and, above all, the hidden pentagram, were interpreted (by the Roman Catholic Church) as signs that it was the fruit that had grown on the tree of forbidden knowledge" and as such the apple also became the symbol of punishment for mankind's gluttonous sin that "leads straight to hell" (Allen, 2003, p. 13). Stewart Lee Allen explains beautifully how the Greek Orthodox Church in turn sees the apple as a symbol of pride and carnal lust; lust and pride incidentally form part of the Catholics' seven deadly sins. Amidst all of this, the Bible is silent on what exactly the forbidden fruit was. But in earlier mythology (in both the Odyssey and Iliad) there is talk of the golden apples in the Garden of Hesperides which are guarded by gods and which can only be had at great peril, although doing so will bring much wealth and wisdom. So here we have two gardens, Eden and Hesperides, and a fruit which is of great value, but is either guarded or forbidden by the prevailing deity. In the one garden it is an apple and unsurprisingly, while the fruit of the second garden is not named, it eventually became an apple too. But according to many tales, apples can be dangerous: taking a bite out of an apple if you are a dark-haired fairy-tale character with "skin white as snow", could lead to an extended and untimely slumber, and unless a suitable prince is found, a curse which will outlast time. Thus, hidden in an apple can be a dooming curse, or it can hold wondrous magic, wisdom, and even eternal wealth, but along the way of mythology and fairy tales there are always the fearful gods and witches who have to be slain.

The history of the apple doesn't stop there. On the Celtic northern side of the Mediterranean, specifically south of the Austro-Italian border, apples were grown for religious ceremonies and apple cider was extensively used for the purpose. Apple cider vinegar today is revered in natural health circles as a powerful metabolic enhancer and follows the logic that cell regeneration is dependent on metabolic health. This slows down atrophy and is believed to counter cellular deterioration, disease, and death (Lax, 2018).

Consider also the symbol of the serpent—the serpent is the seducer; he seduces the woman into eating the apple and she in turn offers it to the man after which they realise both are naked and end up "covering their shame" with fig leaves. Back to the Celtics of southern Italy, where eventually the rivalry between them and the wealthy grape growing northern (and mainly Catholic) people became so bad that the Roman Church banished the apple in 470AD as the Celtic symbol of "evil knowledge" (Allen, 2003, p. 13). Apple, being the symbol of the people and religious system to be overrun by the more powerful Catholic Church, became politics masquerading as religion, and as religion, apple became synonymous with sin until 1452 when Columbus discovered the Americas. He thought the Orinoco River in today's Venezuela to be the entrance to the Garden of Eden, and along with it discovered the "slut-red fruit oozing lugubrious juices and exploding with electric flavours" (known as the tomato of today) and promptly declared it to be the "apple of the paradise", also called the "love apple" (Allen, 2003, p. 18).

Stewart Lee Allen continues with the story in his fascinating book of how, only in the 1700s, Christians started warming up towards this "sinful fruit" when the Italians started using tomato puree in their dishes and as garnish, until St Clement of Alexandria banished sauces as satanic because they enhanced the flavour of foods and thus promoted gluttony (one of the seven deadly sins of Catholicism); but in some quarters the debauchery remained. The tomato was deemed a deadly fruit (note the religious overtone that sin is death). It was only after American Robert Johnson ate a whole one in public in 1820 and lived that the spell was broken and Johnson opened a tomato canning factory, and today we even have ketchup! So, the tomato was redeemed, but in order to be accepted it had to change identity from being the love apple to becoming the tomato.

With the commencement of the post-industrial era, fermented ketchup (which was liable to explode) was outlawed in America's Pure Food and Drug Act of 1906, to be replaced with the cost effective, preservative and additive enriched thick substance that we today know as ketchup. Its' identifying flavour note is *Umami*, which is the note that evokes sensory satisfaction and compels us to eat more. Unsurprisingly, a vast universe of pre-prepared dinners and packaged meals has a tomato base of sorts, and most fast food is served with ketchup. The symbolic power of food is enhanced by the evocation of all the senses; its triggers, emotions, and perceptions are created through mental associations, according to Kats and Weaver (2013).

Symbols of food are often manipulated by the media to give a particular identity to a specific food type, and the tomato continues to feature quite strongly in fast food ads. That juicy, red, luscious tomato that gets sliced, containing its many seeds and excreting its "lugubrious juices" (Allen, 2003, p. 18), sings a song in our unconscious of virility, vitality, and seduction, while our conscious is feebly pointing out that (a) we are seeing the advert after dinner and therefore cannot be hungry, and (b) hamburgers are unhealthy, and the conscious loses the battle. For the use of the tomato in a fast food ad is an act of seduction invoking not hunger, but lust. And here we have powerfully packaged the promise of fulfilment of the three primary needs (food, sex, and safety) in one product—a hamburger, and when some people eat it, they call it "orgasmic". Freudian slip perhaps? Or a very clever play on the archetypical symbolism of the unconscious. And in this with the tomato as symbol the hamburger advertisement and our reaction to it became symbology.

Symbols are often "invented" to control the perception of a particular food product and encourage sales. An example that explains this concept well is bottled water. The perception created by companies is that bottles are filled in natural streams of free-flowing, pure spring water, whereas it is on the contrary bottled in a factory just like any other soda or beverage, according to Martin Lindstrom in *Buyology* (2008). Symbols can also develop rationally, spontaneously, over time, and through everyday usage, and are often called "organic symbols" according to Kats and Weaver (2013). Victor Turner's anthropological properties of symbolism of food can be used to explain this concept:

> Firstly is condensation: many ideas or actions are represented in a single formation. For example, turkey represents the American holiday of Thanksgiving, standing for the family gatherings, feasts, specific menus and football games that commonly occur with the celebration. A second property is unification: symbols link disparate references. The turkey as symbol evokes abundance of natural resources, a romanticized New England heritage, patriotism, family harmony, and the fall of season. The final property of symbols is polarization of meaning: they contain both ideological meanings (representing values, ethos, social norms) and sensory meanings (related to the objective properties of the symbol and representing physical aspects of life), merging these two poles and grounding conceptual references in felt experience. For example, apple pie is an American symbol of both patriotism and maternal nurturing, strengthening the referential power of each yet also lending the emotional associations of each to the other. (Kats & Weaver, 2013, p. 380)

"Food is a rich resource for symbolic communication, expression, and action" (Kats & Weaver, 2013, p. 382).

Julie Parsons's article, "Cheese and Chips out of Styrofoam Containers" (2014) explains how the phenomenon of cooking nutritious food, and the preparation of these foods from scratch, became a symbol of caring and nurturing and indirectly became a distinct symbol of the British middle-class status. Duties that involve planning menus, skilled food preparation from scratch, which at times will involve high wastage amounts, catering for individual dietary requirements and preferences, the sacrificing of valuable time and effort, as well as managing logistics to ensure a family dinner around the table—all symbolise the cultural dissimilarity to the lower classes of British society. Jamie Oliver, a renowned British chef, goes as far as labelling these two distinct classes as the "caring family" which denotes healthy parenting and the "junk family" which consumes pre-prepared food on a regular basis. Convenience foods are indicted by him as tasteless and even careless and symbolise the absence of many qualities that so clearly distinguish the caring aspect of food. He goes as far as saying that the "lack of care is interwoven into a symbolic capital that supposes a lack of time, education, cultural capital, economic capital, and therefore a lack of taste" (Parsons, 2014, p. 6).

She explains that preparation of food from scratch endorses the "good mother" and ensures emotional support of her family. The preparation of the food that has been prepared with great care then signifies the mother's love for her family. This article demonstrates the symbolism that has been recognised under the label of middle-class Britain. Healthy home-made meals have become a symbol of maternal identity and cultural sophistication, care, and love, whereas convenience foods have been demolished to junk status which symbolise an overall lack of many aspects including capital and class.

In further investigation to find evidence for Parsons's conclusions, an article about "poverty and obesity" written by the British Social Issues Research Centre confirmed the above statements (Marsh, 2004). He claims that despite the government's endless campaigns and fight against obesity, obesity is still on the rise. According to him, it's the people that are living on benefits that are more inclined to buy convenience foods as it is a cheaper option. An example given is of mothers who are opting for crisps as a lunch choice, not out of lack of knowledge, but from a lack of options due to money constrains. He also stated that "obesity is linked to social class" where the population is higher in manual and non-skilled professions rather than white-collar and skilled occupations. He urged government to address the underlying issue of poverty, rather than running healthy food campaigns, as the problem is not poor nutritional choices, but lack of affordability of the healthy foods.

Marissa Landrigan discusses in 2014 the symbolism of food in Louisiana, USA by analysing poems written by Sheryl St Germain, a native New Orleans poet. She explores the multifaceted interaction between food, sexual category, and demography. Marissa Landrigan claims in her work that food has been "proven to be one of the most significant symbols of study".

Sheryl St Germain demonstrates how women find their place in society and a sense of belonging through the folklore legacy of food. Through exploring the relationship between women and food, sociologists have discovered that the preparation of food has mainly been the role of the women. Preparation of food is not only a means of survival but it has become "a symbol of women's emotional needs, a rhetoric of protest as well as a language of joy and anguish" (Landrigan, 2014, p. 301). She also emphasises the divergent aspects of how culinary arts are transferred through the ages to their daughters and all females of the society as a symbol of happiness and pleasure.

The history of food: when food was a blessing and fat was fabulous; fat deities united with the divine through food

Marion Woodman (1980) noted that fat was once such a happy state of being. To live off the fat of the land was considered a blessing and in the cultures of the Far East the plump bride is still considered worth her weight in gold. In the oriental cultures of China and Japan in particular, the person exhibiting a round belly is both respected and admired as one who is well grounded in himself. These sentiments are echoed by Richard Klein (1996) who presents the medieval works of Rubens and later of Renoir featuring voluptuous bodies, that would be considered today as morbidly obese, as the epitome of medieval sensuality; he also notes that the thinner bodily forms were commonly featured in artworks dealing with episodes of human misery including the plague and wars. Viktor Frankl (1984) relates how his fellow prisoners in Nazi death camps, immersed in intense misery, would seek temporary escape from their miserable states of mind by discussing their favourite foods when left unobserved by the guards to work within earshot of each other. Throughout most of human history food was seen as a blessing from the gods and as the means to have communion with the gods.

Some of the earliest depictions of human beings' images of their gods show them as fabulously fat, as in Alan Dixson and Barnaby Dixson's work in 2011. They explain that anthropologists noted that only the most important elements of ancient life were immortalised in stone, suggesting that the assumedly obese models who inspired the creation of these figures were either royalty or seen to be embodied with superhuman and divine characteristics. The famous Venus figurines, carved between 20,000 and 30,000 years ago, feature the sort of corpulent thighs, large buttocks, and ample breasts further accentuated by rotund bellies one would associate with a body mass index of well over thirty. In Roman mythology, Venus was the goddess of beauty and love, fertility and sex. The association of plumpness with fertility continued through-out antiquity and was seen as desirable in that it indicated well-being. Hence, most of the goddesses of the period are depicted as rather more matronly than nymph.

Dixson and Dixson go further to explain that the collection of fat goddesses includes the much later Celtic pagan goddess Brigantia whose image is thought to be fashioned in the Roman style after the Roman invasion of the British Isles. As many pagan gods were later Christianised and a recycled version of Brigantia (still fat) was found, appearing as St Brigid, featuring a round face and comfortably padded hips. A reproduction of the sixth-century Norse fertility and love goddess Freya also casts a figure well over a body mass index of thirty, but unlike the similarly fat Greek goddess of love Aphrodite, Freya was also a war goddess. Legend has it that she rode into battle leading the Valkyries and made such an impression that half of the Norse warriors slain in the battle chose to go into her hall in the after-life instead of the hall of the Norse god Odin—the ultimate honour to be bestowed on a goddess by warrior men, as told by Scott Littleton in 2005.

Littleton tells further that the Babylonian goddess Ishtar, although featuring a tiny waist, is shown as having very big thighs, and Hertia, the Greek goddess of the hearth is shown as morbidly obese. Included in the plump goddess collection is Sophia, goddess of wisdom, joined by the rotund Aztec goddess Coatlique and the Anatolian mother god-dess Cybele. Also depicted as obese are Diana of Ephesus and Kuan Yin, the Chinese goddess of mercy, Sekhmet the Egyptian goddess of vengeance, and Luna, the Roman Titaness of the moon who sports a rather heavy pear shape.

The male Silenus, the drunken associate of the Roman wine god Dionysus, was described as the fattest, oldest, wisest, and drunkest of all Dionysus's associates and is lauded in the Orphic hymns as the teacher of the young wine god Dionysus and was said to possess the power of prophesy and special knowledge. Legend has it that Silenus once got lost in Phrygia where he was rescued by peasants and taken to King Midas who treated him kindly. As a gift of gratitude Dionysus offered Midas his chosen reward of being able to turn everything he touched into gold, as related by Luke and Monica Roman (2010).

Food: the gift of the gods

Roman and Roman go on to explain that during ancient times, everything was considered a gift from the gods and food production in particular was seen as a manifestation of divine intervention. Dionysus features as the god of wine and the one who gave nourishment and strength, while Ninkasi, the Mesopotamian goddess of beer was the one who caused dough to rise and it is believed that she inspired the bakers of the day to add sesame seeds and herbs to their bread. In India, as Littleton explains, the goddess of food Annapurna rewarded faithful prayer and sincere worship with rice (*anna* meaning food, and *purna* meaning complete).

The Israelites were kept alive during their forty years wandering in the desert by their God who faithfully supplied manna and quails daily on their way to the Promised Land of Canaan, the land of milk and honey (Exodus, 16:6). Christoph Barth and his associates (1991) explain that manna is still known by the Bedouins who live in the desert of Sin who collect the small white pearls which fall from a plant after the lice have sucked the plant sap and used them as honey to sweeten their food. The manna has to be collected before sunrise, lest the sun melts it and it is eaten by ants. However, when collected early enough in the day, manna has saved many from perishing in the desert both before and after the Israelites. Quails, known by the nomadic desert tribes as good runners but poor fliers (Numbers 11:31 and Psalms 78:26) are easy prey and offer a good survival meal to those lost in the desert. To the Israelites, these daily gifts of food confirmed to them that their Lord was indeed their Shepherd at the very time of their displacement when in their flight they could no longer provide for themselves. Without the divine gifts of manna, quails and water from the rocks, they would not have survived as a nation. Prior to the manna and quails being supplied in the desert, God himself appeared to the Israelites (Exodus 16:6) pointing out that the sustenance would be granted so that the Israelites "shall know that I the Lord am your God (Deuteronomy 29:6 v 12), and "then he gave orders to the skies above and threw open heaven's doors ... he sent them food to their heart's desire" (Psalms 78:23).

The symbology of nectar and ambrosia; honey, manna, and milk in different cultures

Karen Armstrong (2005) tells the story of Tantalus, who was not so lucky. He was the son of Zeus in Greek mythology and was invited by Zeus to eat dinner with the other Greek Gods on Mount Olympus, and then decided to steal the food of the gods, nectar and ambrosia, to share with his mortal friends.

Going further, Tantalus decided to trick the gods into eating human flesh by serving up his own son Pelops, cut into pieces and presented as a stew. For this Zeus himself killed Tantalus and banned him for the entire duration of his afterlife to the underworld Hades, kingdom of the dead. Tantalus's torture was that he had to stand forever waist deep in a pool of water under a fruit tree's branches dangling with ripe fruit. But no matter how hungry or thirsty Tantalus became, there was no relief, for if he bent down to drink the water, it would magically drain away, and if he reached up for the fruit, the branches would lift out of his reach. Displeased gods do not bestow the gifts of food. As Tantalus was already dead, he could not die again of hunger and thirst, but being conscious his punishment was that he had to endure his hunger and thirst for all eternity. Incidentally the English word "tantalise" comes from Tantalus, while a tantalus is a cabinet for decanters featuring a lock.

The nectar and ambrosia, food of the gods, is often portrayed as being produced from the *axis mundi* or what is known as the "Tree of Life", a recurring mythological symbol which finds expression across the world, as well as the mystical connotations of honey (nectar), manna, and milk (ambrosia). In some cultures, nectar was a drink while ambrosia was food, but in other instances the roles reverse. The ambrosia tree of India is known as the tree of Buddha and is also referred to as the tree of wisdom, while the *amrita* (ambrosia) featuring in the Hindu tale recounting the birth of the moon god Chandra drips down from the night skies during a full golden moon as a magical substance onto our plane of existence (Andrews, 2000, p. 158).

The gods of antiquity were generally generous when it came to food. What is known today as vanilla is said to have originated from the Mesoamerican Aztecs and their goddess Xanath in particular, according to Armstrong (2005). Xanath had the misfortune to fall in love with a mortal, but was forbidden to pursue a relationship with him by the other gods. Remembering her love for him, she nevertheless continued to provide his people with vanilla flavouring—which requires no fewer than two species of bees and humming birds for their pollination—for their favourite chocolate drinks and as a consequence, brought them great happiness. Unsurprisingly chocolate is still associated with love today, as explained by Tamra Andrews in her book *Nectar and Ambrosia: An Encyclopaedia of Food in World Mythology* (2000).

She goes on to tell the story of the Native American tribes of the Ojibwa, Cree, Iroquois, and Algonquin who settled the area now known as New England. They had been harvesting maple syrup for thousands of years, and it was seen as the "blood of nature and the symbol of the up-surging life-force of spring" (Andrews, 2000, p. 141), while the Druids and ancient Egyptians chose to swear their oaths by leeks and onions. Each of the layers of these plants' roots was seen as representing a layer of the known worlds, and these multilayered plants were considered a token of eternity (p. 164).

Hazelnuts were associated by the early Europeans with immortality and fertility, and still are far more likely to feature in candies as symbols of romantic love which is an aspect of fertility and served as the symbolic image of the Teutonic god Thor (p. 113).

The symbology of herbs in different cultures

Another romantic ingredient, ginger, was seen as the herb of paradise in the Far East where it was cultivated as flavouring to oils, wine, and teas since antiquity as something that brought one closer to the gods. Ginger is often linked to cinnamon with both being associated with the "solar fire" (the solar fire refers to the divine awakening of the spirit within—similar to the awakening of the *kundalini* in India) and still featuring prominently as key ingredients in magic practices—including love rituals (p. 100).

Not all herbs enjoyed this status. Garlic and its onion relatives were not treated kindly by mythology. The Zoroastrian god of light Ahura Mazda smelled pleasantly while his evil counterpart Ahriman smelled "putrid and rotten" like a garlic bulb (p. 99).

The symbology of grapes in different cultures

Across history, there is no food that rivals the symbolic significance of grapes, and the wine made from them. Known to the Greeks as Dionysus and to the Romans as Bacchus, this god's beauty was second only to Apollo and he discovered wine when he saw animals sucking at grapes to get the juice, as told by Roman and Roman (2010). Dionysus lost no time in fermenting the grapes in a vat to become wine and used the intoxicating effects to recruit a wide range of followers, including the nymphs, the satyrs, and humans who thought that the pleasure they felt when they were drunk gave them a glimpse of what it might be like to be a god. Dionysus was the last of the Olympian gods and also the closest to humans, in that he had a human mother. His gift of wine and the pleasures it brings is still seen as the last and greatest gift from the gods to humanity.

Roman and Roman (2020) explain further that Dionysus was not the only deity with a human mother among the gods. In Christianity wine has become associated with Jesus on two accounts: his turning of water into wine at a wedding so that the guests might continue in joyful celebration at the request of his human mother (John 2:1–11), and as a symbol of sacrifice at the Last Supper where he told his disciples to drink wine in remembrance of him as a symbol of his blood and as the path to eternal salvation (Luke 22:7–23).

The symbology of bananas in different cultures

Terence McKenna tells in 1993 that the banana features in many cultures' mythology, starting with Thailand where *Nang Tani*, a female spirit, guards both her favourite wild banana trees and women. According to the legend, *Nang Tani* would place a curse on the banana trees by haunting the banana groves if men did not treat their wives properly. The banana trees belonged to the men and were the source of their wealth and power. But if they abused this power by oppressing the women, *Nang Tani* would strike at the very source of their power—the banana trees. By guarding the interests of the women, *Nang Tani* in this sense maintained the balance between the duality of nature, the feminine and the masculine principle. In China, the spectral banana maiden is more kind-hearted as she seeks to save lovers who are separated due to non-consenting parents or demonic influences. When she expends too much of her life force, the banana maiden is said to turn into a banana tree. The Burmese myths say one of the very first foods man ate when he was just created were bananas. As he wandered around the forest in search of food, the first man came upon a flock of birds eating the fruit, and took some home which gave the banana its name *hnget pyaw* which literary translates into "the birds told".

The West Africans instead said man was born of the banana tree and it is not unusual for West Africans to bury the placenta of a newborn under a banana tree, which is also a symbolic representation of fertility. Yet it is forbidden to eat its fruits as these are connected to the souls of the children nourishing the tree, but the leaves are used to help women conceive.

The symbology of figs in different cultures

Because fig trees can grow in almost any soil type and climate they quickly dispersed throughout the ancient world and became a central feature in many mythologies, according to McKenna (1993). Tamra Andrews (2000) explains in her book that starting with the Far East, the Buddha found enlightenment under the branches of the bhodi tree, also known as the holy fig, and consequently the tree itself became enlightened.

In Christianity Adam and Eve covered their nakedness in the face of God with fig leaves, while in Greek mythology the tale of Apollo who sent a crow to collect water in a golden goblet is told. According to Roman and Roman (2010), on its way to the water, the crow—a fond lover of figs, saw a fig tree and decided to wait until the fruits ripened. Having eaten her full, she collected the water, which by now was late. On her way back, the crow caught a snake and presented both the snake and the water to the sun god, and claimed the snake was the reason for the delay in getting the water. But the angry Apollo was having none of that and gathered the snake, the crow, and the water and threw them into the sky, and so formed the constellations of Corvus, Crater and Hydra, and since, the Greeks took to offering figs to their gods.

The Romans saw the fig as a source of fertility and named it after the goddess of breastfeeding and fertility, Rumina, due to the fig's milky sap resembling breast milk and the many seeds indicating fertility. The Hindus say that Vishnu was born under a fig tree and that the fig tree was also the mother of Krishna, while Andrews (2000) writes that in Egypt figs were said to be the favourite food of the gods and are often found in burial tombs as gifts to the gods and also to ensure a tasty afterlife for the one entombed.

The symbology of apples in different cultures

Like ambrosia and nectar, apples are strictly reserved in mythology as the food of the gods, and they tend not to view those who attempt to steal apples kindly. While apples are seen as a gift from the gods to man as the symbol of wisdom, fertility, and courage they also serve as the symbol of immortality, and it is this characteristic that renders them strictly confined to the domain of the deities. The tale of the golden apples in the Garden of the Hesperides starts with the Greek goddess Hera, who received the tree that grew the golden apples as a wedding gift from Zeus. She planted it in the middle of the Garden of the Hesperides which was magically hidden and guarded by Ladon, the hundred-headed dragon. The eleventh labour of Hercules was to retrieve the golden apples on the instruction of Eurystheus; the apples once eaten would bestow the gift of immortality on the eater. After much effort to locate the garden, Hercules eventually found it in Illyria where he tricked the titan Atlas to slay the dragon and to retrieve the apples for him, but Hercules's efforts were in vain—the golden apples only worked their magic in Hera's garden.

Similarly, the biblical creation tale told in Genesis features a garden where God communed with Adam and Eve on the condition that they not eat of the fruit of the two trees God planted in the middle of the garden, one representing the knowledge of good and evil and the other eternal life. When Eve, seduced by the serpent eats of the fruit of the tree of the knowledge of good and evil (wisdom) God reacts in wrath, expelling them from the garden which henceforth was to be hidden from men and guarded by angels armed with flaming swords, lest they eat of the tree of eternal life and attain the immortality that would make gods of mere men (Roman & Roman, 2010).

A similar myth is found in the Epic of Gilgamesh, as told by David Ferry in 1992, one of the world's earliest recorded myths that tells the tale of Gilgamesh wanting to consume a magic plant said to bestow immortality. But Gilgamesh's efforts to bring the plant back home were frustrated by the intervention of a serpent who after smelling its sweet fragrance stole it from Gilgamesh and disappeared with the magic plant into the reeds.

Returning to the Greeks, the tale of the Apples of Discord features as its central character Eris, the goddess of discord and strife who brought golden apples to a dinner with the gods of Olympus but said they could only be eaten by the fairest goddess of all. Aphrodite, Hera, and Athena all laid claim to the apples and to prevent further strife, Zeus appointed Paris to declare the winner. Eager to receive his consideration, the striving goddesses showered Paris with gifts, but the day belonged to Aphrodite who presented Paris with Helen, who was so beautiful that her face could launch a thousand ships in the later to be held battle of Troy, to become his wife (Roman & Roman, 2010).

According to Karen Armstrong (2005), in Norse mythology, the goddess Idun guarded the apples which were the source of the gods' immortality, but the trickster Loki started stealing the apples one by one. As the gods began to wither away, they forced Loki to return the apples. Loki turned into a falcon and flew Idun to her hoard where she retrieved them before returning to Asgard where she revived the gods with her apples.

The symbology of pomegranates in different cultures

Roman and Roman (2010) tell that another fruit which was similarly guarded by the gods was the pomegranate—a fruit with a sordid history and jealously coveted by the gods and their followers as a symbol of transformation, seduction, family, and death, and of course—due to its many seeds, fertility. The membrane containing the seeds symbolised marriage and the crown shaped flower became the symbol of both gods and kings. In Greek mythology, the pomegranate started life as a nymph who fell hopelessly in love with Dionysus, the god of wine, theatre, and ecstasy. After hearing from an oracle that one day she would wear a crown, the nymph assumed she would become the wife of Dionysus and in her joy hastened to him, only to be brutally rejected and turned into a tree by the indignant god who had a further insult to offer. To make sure that the oracle's prophesy came true, Dionysus made her flowers into small crowns.

Hera, the goddess of marriage and childbearing, was associated with the pomegranate by followers of her cult who planted pomegranate orchards around all her temples where those who wished for children would come to seek the pomegranates as a blessing. As a symbol of seduction, the pomegranate features in the tale of Persephone and Hades. Hades, god of the underworld, fell madly in love with Persephone, and tempted her to the underworld with a pomegranate. Persephone's mother, Demeter, was so distressed over the loss of Persephone that her sadness caused the earth to grow cold and all the plants to die. The other gods, unwilling to let the earth die demanded that Hades return Persephone, but there was a problem.

The Fates had decreed that anyone who eats or drinks anything in the underworld was condemned to remain there forever, even in the case of someone who was still alive such as Persephone, but a reprieve was found. Hades had only managed to tempt Persephone enough to eat six pomegranate seeds, and that allowed the gods to reach an agreement with the Fates. Going forward, Persephone would be required to spend six months of each year in the underworld with Hades, while her mother Demeter would mourn her absence, and as before the earth would grow cold and plants would die. These became the six months of autumn and winter. But when Persephone was returned at the end of the six months, spring would announce the return of life to the earth. Here, the pomegranate became simultaneously the symbol of the underworld and the cycles of nature.

Rituals with food in different cultures

Roman and Roman (2010) explain that because of food's association with the gods, it remained central to religious practice through the ages as its mediating function in the relations between humanity and their gods endows food with both mysticism and sacred qualities. According to Armstrong (2005), consuming a ritual meal means consuming some element of divinity with the obvious example being the Eucharist where the body and blood of Christ is transubstantiated from bread and wine which is then consumed by the community of the holy to their eternal salvation. Similarly, food offerings to deities were common practice in religious observance and in order to prevent the wrath of the gods, the faithful were required to provide food for the sanctuaries and temples. But the gods have very definite food preferences; in Christianity and Judaism the distinct preference is for the first fruits and lamb without blemish, which had to be consumed in the presence of God by the faithful as thanks offerings to show their joy; while the fat and intestines were to be presented on the altar as burnt offerings. The Egyptian god Set wanted lettuce, while the lord Krishna prefers gifts of butter. But the gods of the Mediterranean wanted stronger stuff, with the Mesopotamian gods demanding beer, while the Greek, Roman,

Egyptian (and Scandinavian) gods all had a distinct liking for wine, as told by Andrews (2000).

He goes on to explain that Ambrosia was the food of the gods on Olympia, and in India, where the Hindu gods' version of ambrosia was called *amrita*, said to be nectar found at the bottom of the ocean, it was a heavenly elixir of immortality. The Hindu goddess Annapurna is shown in Hindu mythology as holding a bowl of porridge and a golden ladle, and would not start eating until all the devotees in her temple had been fed.

Blessings of the gods becomes punishment of unruly people: the symbology of food

As much as the gods of antiquity liked to bless their human follow-ers with food, when humans sought to exceed their bounds in search of immortality, whether stealing golden apples or ambrosia, or eating from a forbidden tree of wisdom, the results were catastrophic. Arm-strong (2005), reflecting on the biblical Adam and Eve, puts it thus: "The loss of the primordial paradise state is experienced as a falling into agri-culture. That is, Adam will actually have to work for his food now," as it was no longer an unconditional gift granted by the gods.

But the gods did not exit the affairs of mankind completely during the agrarian age, as the universal occurrence of harvest festivals and the continued appeasement and food offerings to deities by cultures across the world wishing to be blessed with abundant harvests attests. Similarly, when these harvests were meagre, and famine ensued, up to quite recently in human history mankind believed that it was the result of an offended god who needed to be appeased by repentance so that the plentiful harvests may return.

Early physicians on obesity

It would be amiss to present the impression that the ancient world's adulation of obesity and excess was uniform. The early ancient phy-sicians recognised that obesity was dangerous, with some early con-nections being made between obesity and diabetes. Around 1550 BC Egyptian physicians came to associate excessive urination with over-weight while the symptoms of diabetes are described in early Hindu writings as extreme thirst, high urine output, and the eventual wasting away of the body, but the occurrence of diabetes was only explicitly associated with obesity in the late 1800s, according to Jonathan Wells (2010).

Similarly, obesity did not escape the notice of the Greek physicians with Hippocrates noting the increased mortality associated with obesity, and that "It is very injurious to health to take more food than the constitution will bear, when at the same time one uses no exercise to carry off this excess" (Hippocrates as quoted in Wells, 2010). His remedy? Exercising before meals, consuming a high fat diet which would increase feelings of satiety, but restricting food intake to one meal a day and to stay naked each day for as long as possible, all principles which have since been borne out by modern research on thermodynamics and the principles of appetite regulation and ketosis. Similarly, Herodotus noted the Egyptians' practice of inducing vomiting and to regularly purge themselves believing that such practices aided health, while Galen and Pythagoras recommended restrictions of food intake to control weight gain.

The societal condemnation of obesity was not far behind, with the playwright Aristophanes writing in the fifth century BC that obese men were "bloated, gross, and pre-senile fat rogues with big bellies and dropsical legs which by the gout were tormented" (Wells, 2010, p. 78).

Historical and cultural aspects: achieving communion with the gods—by not eating at all

The early Christians, having defined gluttony as one of the seven deadly sins, also looked at obesity with scorn, starting with Thomas Aquinas's publication of the *Summa Theologiae* in which he describes gluttony as an "inordinate desire … leaving the order of reason, wherein in the good of moral virtue consists" (Aquino & McDermott, 1997, p. 148). Soon, abstinence, the counter-virtue opposing the sin of gluttony came to be seen by the holy anorexics as a way to get close to God; the *anorexia mirabilis* of the Middle Ages referred almost exclusively to a "miraculous lack of appetite" observed mainly in women who would starve themselves in *inedia prodigosa*—the prodigal fast to the point of death in their search for God, as explained by Joan Brumberg in 1989. Rudolph Bell (1987) tells us that unlike its modern cousin, *anorexia nervosa*, which is mainly rooted in the distortion of the body image, *anorexia mirabilis* was but one of many practices of denial which included regular flagellation, the wearing of hair shirts, and celibacy and other practices of penance including sleeping on beds of thorns. The holy anorexics included such characters as Catherine of Siena (1347–1380) who thought of fasting as indicative of female sanctity, humility, and purity, while Caroline Bynum (1987) describes Julian of Norwich's fasting habits as a legitimate means of fellowship with God.

For these holy anorexics, the denial of food was not only about their devotion to God, but they actively sought the separation of body and the immortal spirit. Unlike ancient times when immortality was to be achieved by stealing the food of the gods, the holy anorexics sought to do so by starving their mortal bodies to release their immortal souls in eternal communion with God. Unsurprisingly, they partook of no food with the exception of the Eucharist, but some had rather exotic preferences, with both Angela of Foligno (1248–1309) and Catherine of Siena (1347–1380) drinking the pus from the open sores of the sick they tended, and Angela declaring that the pus was as "sweet as the Eucharist" (Bynam, 1987). Both were also known to have picked the scabs and lice of the sick which they ate.

A psychoanalytic view of the holy anorexics

Bell was quick to point out in 1987 that at least in Catherine's case, not all of her fasting was inspired by holy motives. Catherine's first fast came as a protest to the proposed marriage of her beloved sister Bonaventura who was the one who taught the technique to Catherine in the first place. Bonaventura was known to embark on extended periods of fasting to punish the offensive husband, and would only stop once he showed better manners. If, as the anecdote suggests, these women used to fast as a form of controlling behaviour, then their fasting is not entirely dissimilar to some of the motives underpinning *anorexia nervosa*, an observation underscored by Brumberg in 1989. She noted that the difference between *anorexia mirabilis* and *anorexia nervosa* is not to be found in the motives of those who engage in the behaviour, but rather in that the paradigms for coding the behaviours have changed over time. Bell argues the case differently in 1987. Applying a psychoanalytic lens and placing extensive reliance on Raymond of Capua's biography of Catherine of Siena, originally known as Catherine Benincasa, he concludes that her *anorexia* was less *mirabilis* and more a quest for liberation from patriarchal family and societal dominance and a psychosexual developmental struggle.

Placing great emphasis on her early life and family constellation, Bell noted that she was the twenty-third child who survived at her mother's breast while her twin sister who was sent out to a wet nurse died, leaving Catherine to be weaned very late and with a strong dose of survivor's guilt. This leaves him to conclude that Catherine's frequent reference to maternal imagery was not inspired by the prevailing religious metaphor, but rather was an unconscious recounting of her own early childhood trauma. Catherine sought to avoid sexuality as an adolescent and despite the wishes of her parents who wanted to see her married she joined the Dominican Sisters of Penance after the death of two further beloved sisters. The anorexia soon followed, as Catherine sought out a life of hard penance and solitude which included episodes of intentional scalding and flagellation to tame her "unruly flesh" and earnestly sought absolution for the rest of her life.

According to Caroline Bynum, holy anorexics claimed that their fasting and penance brought them spiritual enlightenment, that "they sat at the delicious banquet of God" and felt "inebriation" with the holy wine and lived in "hunger" for God's eternal presence, and quite a number of these women were said to possess some level of psychic ability (Bynum, 1987, p. 44). They were said to perform miracles like exuding oil through their fingertips, healing with their saliva, and being able to fill empty barrels with wine out of thin air unlike their Saviour who required a bit of water to work with. By the time the advent of the Age of Enlightenment signalled the end of the medieval dark ages, the practice of holy fasting fell out of favour with the Church condemning it as heretical, satanically inspired, and dangerous to the social order.

Gluttony remained a mortal sin with the early nineteenth-century Russian Bishop Brianchavinov declaring that those who pleased their stomachs were hurling themselves over the "precipice of bodily impurity, into the fire of wrath and fury, you will coarsen and darken your mind and in this way you will ruin your powers of attention and self-control, your sobriety and vigilance" (Schimmel, 1997, p. 112), while Lehner and Lehner noted in 1971 that the punishment awaiting those who committed the sin of gluttony was to be forced to eat rats, toads, and snakes in hell for all eternity.

Food and body image as symbols of wealth and power

To the common folk, plumpness still carried considerable value as a sign of prosperity. Peter Stearns noted that thin people were generally regarded with suspicion and seen as ugly. He adds that "to say that Cassius had a lean and hungry look was not a compliment" (Stearns, 1997, p. 12), and points out that until the beginning of the twentieth century, the majority of nutritional interventions were designed to help people gain weight instead of losing it. Similarly, Ogden (1966) also noted that as late as the 1960s thin women in Japan were considered to be unmarriageable while muscular men's prospects were similarly dim as their physique indicated their manual labour occupations.

Stearns wrote that with the advent of the twentieth century came inventions enabling mass production in agriculture which brought a year-round abundance of food, and everyone could live like Mayan royalty, which meant that the plumpness that came with prosperity was democratised. In search of a new status symbol, the elite of the industrial age seized on thinness as a status symbol indicating not only access to better quality food offerings such as unprocessed fruit, vegetables, and lean protein that were considerably more expensive than the highly-processed fare of the masses, but also as a symbol of being better educated.

Culture not only focuses on economic security and prosperity; power also takes on socio-cultural dimensions, and in this context the quantity and quality of food one has access to is vested with a socio-cultural meaning and is indicative of one's wealth and whether one is divinely blessed, according to Aleid Brouwer. Also, consider the case of Hinduism which is generally thought of as a non-material religion, but still features the goddes Lakshmi whom the Hindus workship for wealth and propserity, and whose special dedicated day *Lakshmi puja* remains an integral part in the most liveliest of Hindu festivals, Diwali. Similarly the Bhuddists have their special Bhudda of money featuring the overweight posture and round belly that most Bhuddists associate with material prosperity.

Brouwer elaborates further: the rich as a cultural class consistently use social exclusion and social distancing which includes spatial seperation and other more subtle forms of differentiation to distance themselves from the poor and downtrodden. In this instance the material as evidenced in the accumulation of property, the ability to afford better education or to fund above average consumption are much more than just a means to survival; it is a matter of social status and class identity. This illustrates culture's territorial nature; culture is territorial in that it seeks to differentiate itself from others, whether by race, ethnicity, social class, religion or economic status. It is this imperative for differentiation that drives the materially based cultural dichotomy between the rich and the poor and this materiality is embedded in every culture around the world. This discourse provides support to her observation that the "cultures we produce are the cultures of commodity … for everyday life is the life defined by everyday commodities" (Brouwer, 2008:367) and this defines the materiality of the cultural identity. As being fat was no longer a status symbol of the rich and powerful due to industrial food production, the stigmatisation of obesity began in all earnest as the higher classes sought to differentiate themselves from the rest.

Sander Gilman (2008) notes that "Obesity presents itself today in the form of a 'moral panic'—that is, an 'episode, condition, person or group of persons' that has in recent times been 'defined as a threat to societal values and interests'" (Gilman, 2008, p. 9), and further that "we see obesity as a national rather than an individual problem … not only because of epidemiological evidence, but also because of the meanings now firmly attached to the expansive waistline" (Gilman, 2008, p. 3).

As global obesity is increasing, it is associated with excess weight, ill health, it is regarded morally repugnant and could be socially damaging. Jeffery Sobal and Albert Stunkard suggest that the ridicule of people with obesity remain the last socially accepted form of prejudice. This prejudice begins early in life. Staffieri conducted a study in 1976 of prevailing attitudes among 6-year-old children towards overweight people and found that they described silhouettes of other overweight children as lazy, dirty, stupid and ugly. These findings were confirmed by Phebe Cramer and Tiffany Steinwert in 1998 who found evidence of negative stereotypes towards overweight people in children as young as three years old. Unsurprisingly, these attitudes persist during life, with college students reported to have rated people with obesity as less suitable marriage partners than embezzlers, cocaine users and shoplifters, found by Arthur Vener, Lawrence Krupta, and Roy Gerard in 1982. Similarly, studies by David Klein, Jackob Najman, Arthur F. Kohrman, and Clarke Munro (1982), as well as by Diane Maroney and Sharon Golub (1992) found that healthcare practitioners also tend to hold extremely negative views towards obese patients with physicians and nursing staff reportedly associating obesity with poor hygiene, non-compliance, dishonesty, and hostility. They also saw people with obesity as being more overindulgent, lazier, and less successful at life in general than patients with normal body weight.

In Cramer and Steinwert's study, overweight children held far stronger negative stereotypes towards overweight people than those of average weight. Among adult cohorts, negative attitudes towards overweight people appear to be unrelated to the weight of the respondent (Crandall, 1994), but overweight respondents tend to rate people with obesity as negatively as other respondents suggesting that overweight people themselves associate obesity and overweight with unfavourable character attributes—and more so in early childhood. These anti-fat attitudes also translate into stigma-by-association, as Michelle Hebl and Laura Mannix's study in 2003 illustrated. They asked individuals to rate an average weight male job applicant who was seen either sitting next to an obese woman, or alternatively sitting next to a woman of average weight and noted that in all cases, the job applicant was rated far more negatively by the majority of the respondents when sitting next to the obese woman.

What makes prejudice dangerous, when left unchallenged, is that it tends to translate into active discriminatory behaviour. The findings of Hebl and Mannix illustrate the potential for people with obesity and those they associate with to be evaluated unfairly in employment settings. Indeed, several studies found such discriminatory treatment of people with obesity during all stages of employment from the initial selection as well as discriminatory wage, disciplinary, and promotion practices (Frieze, Olson, & Good, 1990; Pingitore, Dugoni, Tindale, & Spring, 1994; Roehling, 1999). Similarly, Christian Crandall (1994) found that overweight people find themselves victims to weight-related discrimination in educational settings, and Rebecca Puhl and Kelly Brownell (2001) concluded that parents are also less likely to fund the education of their obese children (particularly daughters), which mirrors weight-related discrimination in educational settings that tend to particularly target women.

CHAPTER 5

Concept three: obesity

Early theoretical response to obesity

The historical context of obesity is further explored by Sander Gilman (2008) who points to the nineteenth-century origins of society's concern about childhood obesity, citing Charles Dickens's *Pickwick Papers* of 1837 which describes the morbidly obese servant boy Joe as suffering from "excessive appetite whose corpulent body bore the physical expressions of his monumental stupidity, boundless laziness and moral turpitude" (p. 71). While fat children in Victorian times were seen as character deficient in that they were weak willed, the doctors of the time were more concerned with undernourishment than excess weight, and obesity was hardly seen as a disease until the Viennese clinician Alfred Froehlich described a pubescent boy suffering from a pituitary gland disorder as massively obese and sexually infantile which later became known as Froehlich's syndrome. This allowed the reimagining of fat boy servant Joe to become the poster boy for all cases of pathological childhood obesity.

Adult men similarly saw the stigma of obesity starting with William Banting's *Letter on Corpulence to the Public* published in 1863 while an earlier Verdi opera *Falstaff* told the story of fat men in the fourteenth century seeking a cure for their fatness because they felt socially stigmatised. Similarly, a race connotation was brought to bear on the problem of obesity with Jews being described as a "diabetic race" owing to their alleged inclination to overeat, become overweight and as a consequence, to develop diabetes leading the doctors at the time to observe a link between the "oriental race" and diabetes (Gilman, 2008, p. 111).

The response to this notion came from German-Jewish physician Hilde Bruch who made the link between obesity and family dysfunction—especially bad mothering—in proposing her psychodynamic framework. Instead of dispelling the racial connotation to obesity, by the 1970s the family dysfunction and racial explanations merged in the discourse on obesity pertaining to African American communities. Taking the argument further, Gilman contended that medical research into the demography of obesity tended to perpetuate the idea that race and ethnicity could be precursors to obesity, citing the work of Kenneth Ferraro who found Protestants, in particular Baptists, to be the most obese in the United States, followed by other Christian groups including Catholics and Mormons, while non-Christians (including Jews) were reported to be the least likely to suffer from excess weight.

In making the point that early models of obesity were also "models of race" (Gilman, 2008, p. 125), Gilman draws on Southern American literature including Mitchell's *Gone with the Wind* of 1936 and John Kennedy Toole's *A Confederacy of Dunces* of 1980 to illustrate the racial underpinnings of our understanding of obesity. In *Gone with the Wind* the story of the black Irish is told as they transform to white Irish by rebuilding the South after the Civil War with their supposedly lean bodies, while the tale of ethnic whites' attempt to become fully white is told in *Confederacy*; in this case the effort fails as the characters sink into obesity and ethnicity instead. In contrast, the rising prevalence of obesity in China is ascribed to the invasion of the West with fast food chains such as McDonalds being seen as the primary culprits in the rapid increase of China's "fat little emperors" (Gilman, 2008, p. 138).

In this case, modernisation and the consequent cultural invasion as a result of globalisation is seen as the cause of obesity, as rising incomes and access to American fast food conspire to replicate the American experience of obesity. Yet, in response to the World Health Organization's declaration of a global obesity epidemic in 2001, Gilman noted that our current anxiety about a global obesity epidemic is but "the most

recent iteration of an obsession with control of the body and the promise of universal health" that has characterised modernity (2008, p. 164),
and he observes on his final page that, "Maybe at the end of the day
our desire to control and reform our bodies is what is truly 'modern',
and the obesity epidemic is only proof of our desire to undertake this
quixotic task of absolute bodily control" (p. 174).

An earlier contribution on the cultural obsession with obesity from a
feminist vantage point came from Naomi Wolf in 1991, whose premise is
that the pressure for women to conform to the impossible societal ideal
of beauty and fitness arises from the commercially driven interest por-
trayed in the mass media as a societal response to the increasing power
and social prominence of women. The preoccupation with appearance,
of both genders, leads to unhealthful dietary behaviour and ultimately
compromises women's contributions to and acceptance by society. The
argument is powerfully stated in the introduction to *The Beauty Myth*
as follows:

> The more legal and material hindrances women have broken
> through, the more strictly and heavily and cruelly images of
> female beauty have come to weigh upon us ... During the past
> decade, women breached the power structure; meanwhile, eat-
> ing disorders rose exponentially and cosmetic surgery became
> the fastest-growing specialty ... Pornography became the main
> media category, ahead of legitimate films and records combined,
> and thirty-three thousand American women told researchers that
> they would rather lose ten to fifteen pounds than achieve any other
> goal ... More women have more money and power and scope and
> legal recognition than we have ever had before; but in terms of how
> we feel about ourselves physically, we may actually be worse off
> than our unliberated grandmothers. (Wolf, 1991, p. 10)

Wolf argues consequently that women should have "the choice to do
whatever we want with our faces and bodies without being punished
by an ideology that is using attitudes, economic pressure, and even
legal judgments regarding women's appearance to undermine us psy-
chologically and politically" (1991, pp. 17–18).

Weighing in on the debate, offering a Jungian perspective on the
problem of obesity is Marion Woodman who argues that modern

women have been kept unconscious of their feminine principle as a result of living for centuries in a male-dominated culture, and that this neurosis manifests as obesity. She noted:

> Every woman haunted by obesity knows the agony of looking into a mirror and seeing an owl staring back at her. If she dares to keep looking, she may even see her mermaid's tail. The split between her head and her body is destroying her life and she is powerless to break the spell. (1980, p. 9)

In seeking to find her place in this male world, Marion Woodman contends that women have unknowingly accepted the male values of goal orientation, becoming compulsively driven—but to the feminine soul this is "eating concrete bread which fails to nourish their feminine mystery" (1980, p. 10). This being too much to bear for the feminine essence, the unconscious femininity ends up rebelling by manifesting in a somatic form, and she explains that "the Great Goddess either materialises in the obese or devours the anorexic" (p. 10).

Woodman also explains this by relating the tale of Ophelia, described in *Hamlet* as a father's daughter who grew up without a mother in a court demanding a very specific manner of conduct. In keeping with her social standing, Ophelia fell in love with Prince Hamlet who was destined to take the throne as king. But the affair worked only as long as it was untouched by reality which soon intruded as their "garden" was destroyed having fallen "to all things rank and gross", and here Hamlet realises that Ophelia was no more than a child. She lacked the inner resources to be true to herself, and as a consequence, to him, but as a daddy's girl she continued to play out the role as Hamlet's lover as her father's puppet, and in so doing played false to the man she believed she loved and more importantly—she betrayed the woman she never found within herself. But when her father died and her lover had left, Ophelia went mad and ends up standing in bedraggled dress and weed-braided hair, empty of everything but the demon who possessed her (which Woodman noted, is obesity), and cries "They say the owl was a Baker's daughter. Lord, we know what we are, but we know not what we may be" (Woodman, 1980, p. 15) in reference to an old English legend. The legend tells the tale of Jesus who, passing by the baker's shop and smelling the bread, asked for a piece to eat. The baker, generous of heart, rolled a large piece of dough and put it in the oven to bake bread for Jesus, but his mean-spirited daughter would have none of it. Caught up in the preparations and her own fantasies of the Christmas Day to come, she misses the reality present-ing as a beggar at the back door. She believed the piece of dough too large, and reduced it to a much smaller size. But after all, it was the Saviour's dough, and it swells to an enormous size upon which the daughter responds in horror—the mystery rejected at the back door shows up as the monster in the centre of the room. Overcome by the dough, Jesus turns the daughter into an owl as punishment for her stinginess.

Being turned into an owl is not without symbolic meaning. In Greek mythology, the owl was Athena's bird symbolising Athena's affin-ity with darkness. Like Ophelia, Athena was also a daddy's girl, who sprung from her father's forehead after he swallowed her pregnant mother. Shakespeare presents the immature Ophelia as a little walk-ing owl, simultaneously bewitched by her unconscious feminine while held captive by her father's expectations and what "they say". As a result, she misses life and love and the present as she never completed the development work of finding her own voice, her own identity, and her own body. As she dies and her body is swept away by the brook, the "waters of the unconscious to which she is native and endued swallow her" (Woodman, 1980, p. 14). Woodman concludes that "Only by dis-covering and loving the goddess lost within her own rejected body, can a woman hear her own authentic voice" (p. 10).

Wolf's contribution was not received uncritically, with Christina Sommers pointing out in 1995 that Wolf's historical analysis was flawed and that her statistic claiming that 150,000 women died of anorexia each year was inaccurate. The critique of statistical overreach was further supported by Casper Schoemaker in 2004 who found that the anorexia statistic quoted by Wolf could likely be divided by eight to arrive at a more realistic estimate.

Yet Richard Klein (1996) offers support to Wolf's main premise regarding the pressure to conform to the societal ideal of beauty in that the combination utopianism, moralism, and modern consumer culture conspire to make it extremely painful for those who do not conform to the prevailing norms of beauty and acceptability to simply be them-selves, arguing that the beauty and diet industry is so intense that it causes not only material denial as people continue to follow extreme diet and beauty regimes, but the very denial of the soul. Klein writes:

My position is this, even if fat is unhealthy, which it is and it isn't, for the vast majority of people, it's probably healthier than the alternative. The alternative is dieting, compulsive exercise, hyper-vegetarianism, diet pills. My opinions start from the *a priori* premise that administering any powerful drugs to a large population over a long period of time is not good for public health. (1996, p. 87)

The public condemnation of obesity

As mentioned earlier, a great concern of the World Health Organization is that obesity rates are relentlessly on the upsurge, and public health systems are coming increasingly under pressure due to the costs of caring for people who suffer the lifestyle diseases associated with obesity. What gives legitimacy to the public outrage is that it is public health systems that bear the costs, and as such, private lifestyle choices impose public consequences. Globally the World Health Organization reported that in 2015, 1.9 billion people were overweight, of which 600 million were classified as obese; and obesity is rising. However, the problem is not universal—some countries such as Japan—which maintained an obesity rate of around 3% from 2004 to 2014—have not fallen prey to rising obesity levels.

Where obesity and the public condemnation thereof abounds, the weight loss market is booming. According to Markets and Markets (2016), the global weight loss market was estimated to be worth US$ 586.3 billion in 2014 and had an average compound annual growth rate of 10% from 2009 to 2014. Weight loss is profitable business—statistics show that fewer than 2.5% of people who manage to regain control of their weight maintain their weight loss over the long term—and these are the repeat customers of the industry. Often, these cases include people who have managed substantial weight loss as a result of prolonged caloric restrictive diets and exercise regimes, and explanations on why they eventually pick up the weight despite showing considerable self-restraint over these prolonged periods are lacking (Coulston, 1998; Field et al., 2003; Goodrick & Foreyt, 1991).

The medical evidence outlining the dire health consequences associated with obesity, which is what much of the public condemnation of obesity is based on, has not gone unchallenged. Paul Campos argues that the "current barrage of claims about the supposedly devastating medical and economic consequences of excess weight is a product of greed, junk science and outright bigotry. It blows the whistle on a witch hunt masquerading as a public health initiative by exposing the invidious cultural forces that encourage us to hate our bodies if they fail to conform to an arbitrary and absurdly restrictive ideal" (2004, p. xvii).

Campos evaluates four central claims made by medical research on obesity;

(a) That obesity is assuming epidemic proportions in almost all high- and middle-income countries (World Health Organization, 2003, p. 61). Allison Hedley and her associates note that for this to be true an exponential pattern in the growth of obesity must be observed which is not borne out by the available data which instead show that the majority of those classified currently as obese and overweight are currently at weight levels slightly higher than those maintained a generation ago, and further that adult and childhood body mass index may have ceased to increase (Hedley et al., 2004).

(b) Catherine Flegal and her associates dismissed the claim that overweight and obesity are major contributors to mortality by citing studies indicating that no increased risk of early mortality is observed until one reaches a body mass index of 30, and that within the US context it was found that those with a body mass index of below 25 in fact faced a higher risk of premature death than those above it (Flegal, Graubard, Williamson, & Gail, 2005).

(c) Similarly, the claim that higher than average adiposity is pathological and a primary cause of disease is dismissed by the authors claiming that very little evidence show exactly how adiposity causes disease and that to the contrary the claim that adiposity is itself pathological is not supported by interventions aimed at reducing adiposity only (S. Klein et al., 2004). Where health improvements do occur, the authors claim that these arise from the lifestyle changes associated with weight loss, not the reduction in adiposity itself.

(d) The claim that long-term weight loss is medically beneficial in that it reduces early mortality is dismissed on the basis that it is untested. The authors argue that for such a claim to be established it needs to be tested. It would require significant long-term weight loss in statistically significant cohorts, a quest rendered impossible by the low number of people who manage to lose weight over the long term. In particular, they vehemently criticise the pursuit of an untested long-term health goal by the current life-threatening means of weight loss surgery, diet drugs known to induce adverse consequences, fad diets, and chronic weight cycling. Edward Gregg, Robert Gerzoff, Theodore Thompson, and David Williamson point in 2004 to data from the US National Health Survey which shows that people with obesity including those suffering from type 2 diabetes who tried to lose weight and failed suffered a mortality rate no greater—and in some cases less—than those who did succeed in their weight loss efforts. This study also associated weight loss with a mortality risk ratio of 3.36 and weight cycling with a risk ratio of 1.83 (Diaz, Mainous, & Everett, 2005), while finding that people with obesity of stable weight had no increase in mortality.

Concluding his review, Campos and associates dismissed the notion of an obesity-driven health crisis in 2006 and suggested that the war on fat is driven more by political factors, profit motive, and culture than any legitimate concern about the risks increasing body weight may pose to public health.

Similar to Klein who claimed that the growing emphasis of dieting and exercise was the root cause of the rapid increase in overall levels of obesity, Campos and associates argue that the damage wrought by the war on fat goes far beyond its tendency to expand our waistlines. Historically most attempts to marginalise and shame some disfavoured class of people have focused on some minority group or another. The war on fat in America is unique in that it represents the first concerted attempt to transform the vast majority of the nation's citizens into social pariahs to be pitied and scorned until weapons of mass destruction can be found that will rid them of their shameful condition. As we shall see, this is a phony war, fought against an enemy that cannot be defeated, because he does not exist. (2004, p. xvii)

So pervasive is the notion of the ideal body weight that Campos and his associates (2006) noted that the majority of dieticians in the US were victims of eating disorders and consequently prone to the very thinking patterns that motivates them. They ascribe this to the prevalence of what he terms the "anorexic lens" and claims that the proposed ideal body mass index of 21.9—a definition that would make a woman of average height weighing 128 pound "fat"—and the emulation of ultra-lean models and movie stars in contemporary culture as forms of anorexic ideation. The consequence of this anorexic ideation for Campos and associates is an eating disordered culture, one that obsesses about obesity and is characterised by an intense loathing of body diversity and neurotically oscillating between "guilt-ridden bingeing and anorexic starvation"—a culture that has become pathological in its fearful loathing of food, pleasure, and life itself, and further describes the culture of diet as one of perpetual dissatisfaction; and he concludes that:

> The rejection of the war on fat is based on a simple principle: that tolerance toward an almost wholly benign form of human diversity is the least we should expect of ourselves, if we wish to lay claim to living in a civilised culture. The war on fat is an outrage to values— of equality, of tolerance, of fairness, and indeed of fundamental decency towards those who are different. (2004, p. xvii)

Nonetheless, Campos and associates' critique of the science of obesity has not gone unchallenged. Soowon Kim and Barry Popkin (2006) published a comprehensive critique of Campos and his associates' argument by offering an extensive overview on the epidemiology of overweight and obesity. Their first argument is that Campos and associates cited the literature supporting his assertions rather selectively and point out that data from around the world suggest radical increases in obesity levels in contrast to their argument that these increases were subtle at best. Similarly, Kim and Popkin point out that the adverse health effects of obesity are real.

While Campos and his associates are correct in describing the relationships between the degree of obesity and the consequent health effects as complex, June Stevens and her associates (1998), amongst others, made these links quite clear and explicit. Kim and Popkin point out that at the heart of the debate raised by Campos and associates is the issue of how obesity fits into the pathway linking weight with health outcomes. They noted that considerable progress was made in research on the pathways, risk factors, and mechanisms linking obesity to adverse health and that they ignored this pathway. The authors conclude their analysis by noting that recent research has yielded strong evidence supporting the prevailing medical view that obesity and overweight is indeed linked to certain cancers, increased hypertension, diabetes, stroke, and coronary heart disease.

Obesity in the context of the social construct and people's relationships with food in the unconscious

What is fascinating about this debate is not so much the merits of conventional medical research regarding the adverse health impacts arising from overweight and obesity, but the very shrillness of this raging debate. Obesity in the social mind is more than just the physical outcome of an unhealthy eating pattern; it has become a social construct indicative of socioeconomic class and educational attainment, and on an individual level, the quality of one's character.

The relationship with food is core to the problem, both biologically and evolutionarily as a survival issue, and, due to cultures, habits, which turn food into social discourse and a medium for sustaining relationships. Therefore, the relationship with food is an unconscious matter. Eating behaviour and reactions to food are functions of cultural conditioning, exposure to food, socioeconomic class, and personal experiences—and these tend to be embedded in the unconscious, often laden with emotional content (Bruce-Mitford, 2008).

Jung described the collective or transpersonal unconscious as a level of unconscious shared collectively with other humans and which comprises latent memories of our evolutionary, cultural, and historical (or ancestral) past. He concluded that "the form of the world into which a person is born is already inborn in him as a virtual image" (Jung, 1953, p. 188). Jung referred to these ancestral images as archetypes which are images and thoughts that have universal meanings across cultures. Archetypes are expressed in dreams, literature, art, or religion, and Jung explained that the reason why some symbols have the same meaning across different cultures was because they derive from archetypes shared by the whole of humanity. Hence, Jung believed that the basis for human behaviour lies in our primitive past which directs the human psyche.

Narratives' influence on the human psyche. The story of *Hansel and Gretel*: an example of the rich symbolic meaning of food conveyed over generations

To illustrate the above-mentioned concept, consider the rich symbolism in the Germanic tale by Grimm and Pacovska that was written in 1812 of *Hansel and Gretel*, the children of a woodcutter. The tale starts off with the children's stepmother who demanded that their father leave them in the woods. There was famine in the land and according to the stepmother the children ate too much and she wanted to ensure that she and the husband did not starve to death. The woodcutter initially opposed the plan, but eventually relented. However, their discussions were overheard by the children, and Hansel prepared for the inevitable by going out that night to collect white pebbles. The next day, as planned, the stepmother and father took the children into the woods. Hansel left a trail of white pebbles which became luminous in the moonlight to help the children find their way home, much to the consternation of the stepmother.

Food was scarce, and the parents decided to take the children to the woods again, but this time, they locked the door and Hansel could not gather pebbles to guide them home. Instead, on his way out, Hansel grabbed a piece of bread and left a trail of breadcrumbs to guide them home. Despite Hansel's plan, the children could not find the trail for it was eaten by the birds, and they were lost in the woods. After hopelessly wandering around for days, they eventually spotted a white bird in a clearing who led them to that ultimate children's paradise and sensual temptation—the witch's cottage that was made of gingerbread (in earlier versions sweet bread) and all kinds of sweets imaginable. The windows were made of translucent sugar, the door handle was a sugar cane, and everywhere they looked, sweets abounded. In their hunger, the children started eating the roof. The door opened to reveal a hideous old hag who lured them inside with promises of soft beds and delicious food. This seduction is echoed in other children's stories starting with the nursery rhyme by Mary Howitt published in 1829 and later parodied by Lewis Carroll's "Lobster Quadrille" in *Alice's Adventures in Wonderland* (as written by Martin Gardner in *The Annotated Alice*, 1998).

> Will you walk into my parlour?" said the Spider to the Fly,
> 'Tis the prettiest little parlour that ever you did spy;
> the way into my parlour is up a winding stair,
> and I've got many curious things to show you when you are there.
> (Howitt & DiTerlizzi, 2002, p. 2)

The witch was a bloodthirsty hag who locked Hansel in a cage the next morning and Gretel became her house slave. In planning to eat Hansel, she started fattening him up. Hansel in turn fooled the blind witch, by offering a bone instead of his finger every time she checked up on his weight gain. Eventually the witch lost patience and decided to eat him anyway. The witch prepared the oven for Hansel, and decided to eat Gretel as well. To lure Gretel into the oven, she coaxed her to lean over and open the oven so that she could feel whether it was hot enough for cooking. But Gretel was no fool; she sensed the witch's intent and feigned ignorance. The exasperated witch was forced to demonstrate how to check the oven, upon which Gretel pushed her into the oven and freed Hansel. Together, the pair discovered a vase full of precious stones in the witch's house and put the jewels into their clothing. They set off on their way home, assisted this time by a white swan who ferried them across the lake. Upon their arrival at home they discovered that the evil stepmother had died and that their father spent his days in mourning the loss of his children. Happiness returned to the house, and thanks to the witch's treasure they were rich and lived happily ever after.

According to Dee Ashliman (1998), the story is said to have originated during the Great Famine of 1315–1321 in Europe. In this time, it was common practice for desperate people to abandon young children or to resort to cannibalism (Tatar, 1987). In the Grimm and Grimm version of 1884, the mother was the children's biological mother.

The tale offers richness in symbolism and food in particular serves the central symbolic role. It was the lack of food that served as the justification for abandoning the children. It was the lack of food and the children's hunger that kept them awake at night so that they overheard the parents' plans. However, their hunger saved them—having overheard the plans; they knew to collect stones and bread so that they could return to their home. But then food became the dangerous seducer as the children were attracted to the witch's edible house—the baited trap that led them into captivity and slavery. Their hunger rendered them vulnerable to the witch's promises and led them into the house. Food became the tormentor as the witch sadistically used it as a means to fatten Hansel up, so that he could become her next meal. But food is also the decoy as Hansel, surrounded by a feast of plenty, had a bone to offer instead of his finger to deceive the witch and put off his inevitable demise. In this story food is a catalyst, a protector, seducer, and abuser—it divided a family leading to the abandonment of the children, it led the children into a trap, but it also sustained them. And herein one finds summarised the very essence of our deeply conflicted relationship with food, as described by Maria Tatar's writings of 1987.

The rich symbolism of the tale does not end with the food—for it is also a tale of transformation, of coming of age. The forest is a recurring image in European folklore; it is a supernatural world where the unexpected and magical can happen. In Jungian psychology, the forest is a metaphor for the feminine principle which represents the unconscious. As the leaves block the sun's rays (the sun representing the masculine principle), the forest world is often darkened, and symbolising the dangerous side of the unconscious—that place where reason is destroyed (Cirlot, 1971; Matthews, 1986).

By identifying the father as a woodcutter, a class element enters the story. The woodcutter is the lowest paid occupation, and as the family eventually triumphs over the witch and the poverty, the tale—according to Jack Zipes's writings of 1997—represents a triumph of the poor over the richer classes represented by the witch. Because she is richer (with a vase full of jewels), she has food in store which she uses to lure the children. Zipes noted that the killing of the witch is indicative of the hatred the peasantry felt for the aristocracy who they saw as hoarders and oppressors; and by relieving the witch of her jewels, the family could live happily ever after.

The names of the children carry no special significance, as Hansel and Gretel were very common names representing everyman at the time. The famine, added by the Brothers Grimm in the fifth edition of the tale, is used as a justification for the parents abandoning the children (Rölleke, 1988). According to Hans Dieckman, Bruno Bettelheim, and Boris Matthews, the bread in the story is used as a symbol of transformation in that it illustrates the children's journey from childhood to adulthood, but the symbolism extends to several levels. First, bread is the food of the poor, but it is also seen as the basis of daily substance (Matthews, 1986), and as such the struggle to provide bread for the children illustrates the family's struggle for survival and their extreme poverty.

The abandonment of the children in the tale introduces the distinctly Freudian concepts of fear of abandonment and oral greed (Hoyme, 1988). Freudian analyst Bruno Bettelheim noted that children fear abandonment by their parents, but simultaneously they are also orally greedy and fear starvation by their parents if they are overly greedy—this tale to an extent addresses these fears, but the opposite themes of parental abuse and poverty are also present. Similarly, being left alone in the woods represents both the loss of security for the children and the abandonment of previously held truths (Heuscher, 1974). In Hansel and Gretel's world, women are depicted as dangerous: the stepmother who agitated for their eventual abandonment and a witch who seduced them and ultimately wanted to consume them. The image of the evil stepmother is associated with images of jealousy, selfishness, and cruelty in fairy tales (Olderr, 1986). And as Marie-Louise Von Franz and Kendra Crossen (1970) noted, in masculine psychology the evil stepmother represents the unconscious in a destructive role.

Von Franz and Crossen explain further that as destructive as the stepmother figure is, it was her actions that drove the protagonists into the situation that allowed them to discover their strengths and showcase their best qualities—for in the battle with the stepmother, the protagonist prevails in fairy tales. In contrast, the father figure began by being the voice of mercy in that he opposed the stepmother's calls to lead the children into the woods initially, only to return later as the ineffective and weeping father who mourned the loss of his children, and as such, the tale carried strong patriarchal overtones. This is also reflected in Hansel's role at the beginning of the story where he was the one to collect the pebbles that allowed them to find their way home, and he was the one protecting his sister. But then he landed in captivity, and Gretel ended up slaying the witch, and setting her brother free.

The moon of course, represents light, while the white pebbles symbolise justice; the ancient Greeks saw a vote using a white pebble as an indication that the voter felt the accused was not guilty, while white pebbles were often placed at grave sites to ensure the rebirth of the spirit of the one entombed there (Olderr, 1986). Dieckman and his co-authors have a different interpretation; the white pebbles symbolised the children's rigidity to change. In the second instance, Hansel relied on bread crumbs to point the way home. As Bettelheim (1976) noted from the Freudian perspective, starvation anxiety was the driving force for Hansel to want to go back home, and overcome by starvation anxiety he can only think of food as his solution to find his way out from the predicament abandonment presents.

The pigeons in the tale represent a death omen in one sense, as a pigeon—especially a white pigeon flying towards a house—is indicative of a death (Opie & Tatem, 1989); and as the story revealed, the white pigeon indeed led the children to the house they were supposed to die in. Pigeons can also be associated with a desire to return home: homing pigeons are prized for their ability to find their way home.

Birds in general are dominant in the tale—the birds ate their crumbs, it was a bird that led them to the witch's house, and it was a bird that provided the children's final escape by ferrying them across the water (Tatar, 2002). According to Steven Olderr (1986), birds are often used as symbols for air, wind, time, immortality, the feminine principle, spirit, love, freedom, aspiration, and prophesy. Von Franz and Crossen noted in 1970 that following an animal into a forest represents being led to a confrontation in the unconscious. In this case the bird is white, which according to Dieckman and associates (1986) signified that a positive outcome will result.

The witch's cottage was made of gingerbread—cake is a symbol of the rich, a symbol of feasting and plenty (Olderr, 1986), and the sugar signifies excess in the midst of the famine which led to the children's abandonment in the first place. But the witch is a universal symbol across cultures (Leach & Fried, 1949) and in Jungian psychology the witch is the physical manifestation of evil which eventually consumes itself; as such the witch also symbolises the destructive power of the unconscious. Jack Zipes noted in 1997 with interest that the children never blame their parents for their abandonment in that in returning with their bounty they have every intention of sharing it with them; the witch in contrast, with her greed and treasures, represents the feudal system which the children overthrow. She is also a cannibal, guilty of transgressing one of the most universal taboos in the world, which makes her especially hideous and evil, and the demonic fury that possesses her is evidenced in her red eyes that cannot see far.

Eyesight is associated with mental clarity, suggesting the witch was so depraved that she no longer possessed control of her faculties, and so enraptured was she at the thought of eating both children that she lost sight of the child in front of her who would push her into the oven. Jungian analysts perceive this action as both a symbol of birth and transformation (the oven as a womb), according to Dieckman, Bettelheim, and Matthews (1986), as it is an ally in the form of a destroyer, and a trap as seen as a symbol of the witch's or mother's womb. Derek Brewer (1988) explains that by going back into the womb, the womb becomes a tomb in that it prevents the growth of the individual who remains in it, or returns to it as an act of regression.

Olderr (1986) explains that the finger is the force of the unconscious that can emerge despite the efforts of the conscious, but Hansel was careful not to show it to the witch, using a bone to deceive her instead.

The bone itself is fraught with symbolic meaning as it represents the indestructible part of man. At this point in the story Hansel's life is in grave danger, but the trickery and symbolism of the bone suggests that he will survive. Joyce Thomas (1989) similarly noted the trickery associated with the bone which represents starvation and deprivation—the central themes of the tale. Trickery is the means by which one slays witches and dragons and evades ogres in fairy tales, but to do so the trickster must experience and accept evil within him- or herself (Jung's shadow), because by embracing evil (Hansel becoming a dishonest trickster, Gretel becoming a murderess) the witch can be overcome (Mario, Kast, & Riedel, 1992).

Burning often occurs in fairy tales as a symbol of purification, and the witch's burning in the oven is no exception (Luthi, 1976). Similarly, Mueller, as cited in Bottigheimer's writings of 2014, noted that the punishment of witchcraft in medieval Europe was to burn them alive. Donna Napoli retells the tale of *Hansel and Gretel* from the witch's perspective in 1995, which also illustrates the purification by burning motif. According to her iteration, the witch started out as a wise old hag who was skilled in the healing arts. Her skills as a midwife in particular were in high demand and she worked tirelessly to serve God, and to benefit her beloved daughter Asa—often preferring as payment things of beauty Asa would desire such as the perfect hair bow and other trinkets. But then her neighbour, Bala (a reincarnation of the God Baal), convinces her that she would be able to better serve Asa by working for the rich, and at this point the wise old hag becomes the evil sorceress (note the class motif here). Eventually the demons trick the sorceress by presenting her with a beautiful ring for the now grown Asa, and the sorceress succumbs. Now fallen she flees to a foreign land where she becomes the witch of *Hansel and Gretel*'s story, condemned to demonic possession manifesting as cannibalism. She builds her beautiful sweet encrusted gingerbread cottage in the woods that would have delighted her beloved daughter Asa, in remembrance of her. The sweet encrusted house which literally encases the witch in all of the temptations of the flesh serves as a testament of the witch's ability to resist temptation, and this temperance renders the sweets sacred by virtue of not being eaten.

The witch must live alone so that she can resist the temptation given by the demons to all witches—the compulsion to devour young children; and at this point Hansel and Gretel enter the magic circle. This tale, too, is rich with symbolism: the intelligent, self-reliant woman who chooses a path of piety and resists vanity and pride until she is seduced by material longing, not for herself, but for her daughter. Once having succumbed to the demons that lured her, she continues to resist them by isolating herself in the woods and leaving her daughter so that she might not commit that ghastly sin of all witches—eating a child. In Napoli's version, the desire for salvation is made manifest by the witch wilfully allowing Gretel to push her into the oven, and finds redemption in again offering her own life for the child's—first Asa and then Gretel. In the flames, the witch can at last know that she is saved.

In the obvious overtones of denial and penance that were such a central feature in the holy anorexics' search for redemption that has echoes in this tale, the anorexic manifests as a witch, damned by demonic possession; her compulsion to devour the lives of children (as metaphor for the future and purity), lies at the root of her isolation. But for her strength, intelligence, and piety, she finds her final redemption in sacrifice. The circle drawn around the witch's house holds the demons at bay—as long as both witch and children do not cross its bounds, and the perimeter of the circle represents the limits of self-denial. When these limits are breached, the demons regain their power over the witch, and in this rendition of the tale it is the ability to resist the profane (eating of children) that sets apart the profound (the eventual self-sacrifice of the witch by allowing Gretel to push her into the oven so that the witch may find salvation and Gretel be saved) (Napoli, 1995).

Returning to the original version of the story, the children are justified in their taking of the witch's treasure because she wanted to kill them. They then proceed to cross the lake. Bettelheim (1976) relates the crossing of a body of water to the baptism rite, indicative of the transcendence of the children's consciousness into a higher level of existence. In psychoanalysis, water is the symbol of the feminine and the unconscious (Matthews, 1986). The children cross the water by being carried separately on the back of a white swan. Davies (1996) relates the swan to a symbol of maternal replacement since swans, along with geese and ducks, represent the feminine in Germanic tradition. The swan takes the children home whereas their stepmother abandoned them.

The children being carried across separately also illustrates their newfound maturity as individuals. Gretel no longer needs Hansel to hold her hand and can cross the lake without his help. Similarly, Hansel, having been saved by Gretel, crosses separately as he transcends his captivity and enters maturity, as interpreted by Bettelheim. Upon their return home, the children hear the stepmother has died and the coincidence of her death with that of the witch who died in the oven gives rise to the suggestion that the stepmother and the witch are metaphorically the same woman (Brewer, 1988).

The motif is echoed in a Slavic folk tale which tells of an evil step-mother (also the wife of a woodcutter) who sends her daughter into the woods on the pretext of going to borrow a lamp. The evil stepmother turns out to be *Baba Yaga*—a deformed witch commonly depicted as standing on chicken legs, who similarly has a taste for children. But she is not straightforward: occasionally evil, sometimes helpful, but mostly ambivalent, and as is the case with Napoli's witch in his writings of 1995, Baba Yaga is not a singularly evil figure; in both cases, evil and good are not mutually exclusive, but rather coexisting concepts. This duality references the third archetype identified by Jung and referred to as the shadow (similar to Freud's id), which is the animal side of the human psyche and the source of both humanity's creative and destructive energies (evil). In contrast, the persona presents as the socially conformant, acceptable face of the personality (good). The self was identified by Jung as the final archetype and is the source of unity in experience. The ultimate developmental aim, according to Jung, is for every individual to achieve a unified state of selfhood or, put differently, the embrace of the shadow which requires the acceptance of the coexistent duality of good and evil. For Jung pathology derives from the individual's progressive alienation from his instinctual foundation and the path to healing requires the individual to reconnect with that foundation.

CHAPTER 6

Concept four: the collective unconscious (the Jungian perspective)

B oth Freud's and Jung's work focused extensively on the unconscious and the extent to which it drives pathological behaviour. For Freud, the unconscious was personal and for Jung it was both personal and collective. Nevertheless, the language of the unconscious is symbols, expressed through dreams, embodied in myths, and both authors identified the archetypes. Like Freud, Jung also believed that the healing task was to make the unconscious conscious. Freud perceived the unconscious as the seat of unresolved personal trauma; by bringing the unconscious trauma to the conscious, personal trauma could be resolved. Jung believed thatby making the unconscious conscious, trauma is resolved, but more so a broader developmental task is served, through the processes of transformation and individuation.

The validity of Jung's contribution illustrated by quantum theory

Diogo Ponte and Lothar Schäfer explained in 2013 that Jung's ideas of the collective unconscious, the archetypes, synchronicity, and individuation were presented in a world dominated by Newtonian physics, the material universe of classical physics. As a result, the concept never found mainstream favour at the time and was vehemently criticised to the point of dismissal.

Ponte and Schäfer explain further that these ideas were not entirely new; in the nineteenth century Hegel taught that the primary structure of the universe was "absolute spirit": the spirit that *is* everything, in that it creates everything including thinking and being, the real and ideal, the human and divine, all of which are one. Similarly, the ancient Indian sages taught that while one could find consciousness in a thousand human minds, there is only one consciousness which they termed the cosmic consciousness. The Indian sages termed this *Santana Dharma* and the sixteenth-century philosopher Agostino Steuco introduced the concept to Western philosophy as perennial philosophy. The history of human thinking is characterised by recurring truths that are so fundamental that they keep reappearing. In the worlds of quantum physics and Jungian psychology, these truths reappear as synchronicity which suggests that the human mind is a mystical mind in that it is connected with a cosmic background that has mind-like properties, in other words, a cosmic mind, according to Menas Kafatos and Robert Nadeau in 1990.

The contribution of quantum physics was that of discovering a nonempirical realm of the universe that was shown to consist of forms, not matter as classical physics suggested. These invisible forms are real because they have the potential to appear in the physical world and act in it; and it is this property of forms that gives rise to the central thesis of quantum physics: the empirical world emanates out of a cosmic realm of potentiality. The forms of the cosmic realm appear either as physical structures or things in the external world, or as archetypical concepts in our mind (Ponte & Schäfer, 2013). Similarly, in a quantum world the evolution of life is not the process of adaptation of species to their external and physical environment, as the material universe proposed by Newton, Darwin, and others would suggest, but rather the adaptation of our minds to the increasingly complex forms that exist in the cosmic potentiality (Eddington, 1939).

Seen in this context, Jung's proposition that our psyche is guided by archetypes, a system of forms in the quantum sense, which while they do not carry any mass or energy are nevertheless powerful and which are invisible but nonetheless real, does not seem that far-fetched anymore.

Jung described the archetypes as existing in a "psychic system of a collective, universal, and impersonal in nature" (Jung, 1969, pp. 43–44). It is out of this system that Jung wrote "the invisible can appear in our mind and guide our imagination, perception and thinking" (Jung, 1969, p. 44). Jung's views found substantial support in the discoveries of quantum physics which in itself came as a shock to the prevailing worldview in Western science, as it exposed the fundamental errors of classical physics; what was thought of as the material world was in fact non-material, consisting of non-material forms, but real for they have the potential to appear in the physical world and to act on it (Eddington, 1939).

This is what forms the realm of potentiality in the physical reality and all empirical "things" have their origin in this realm of potentiality. More so, the forms of the cosmic potentiality are patterns of information representing as waves, thought-like in nature, and they converge much like the thoughts in a person's consciousness (Ponte & Schäfer, 2013). The implication is that the universe appears to be an undivided wholeness in which all matter and life are interconnected, which means that consciousness is a cosmic property and because it is an interconnected universe, all individual minds are connected to the cosmic mind. This coincides exactly with the central premise of analytical psychology proposed by Jung. The discovery of a realm of non-material forms which exist in the interconnected cosmic reality as the basis of what we perceive in the physical world supports the acceptance of Jung's archetypes. The archetypes are indeed real *forms* which appear in our unconscious out of the cosmic realm, or as Jung termed it, the collective unconscious, where they are stored and manifest as matter in the physical world.

Quantum physics confirmed Jung's view "that it is not only possible, but fairly probable even, that psyche and matter are two different aspects of the same thing" (Jung, 1969, p. 57). Writing singly, Schäfer describes in 2013 the concept in quantum physics as follows. At the foundation of the visible world are entities which appear as elementary things when we interact with them. Left alone, these elementary things revert to their natural state which is not matter, but waves. As waves, they have no mass as matter does, and they become pure forms—patterns of information; something more "thought" like than "thing" like.

Since waves are extended in space, a wave has no specific position in space, but many potential positions, and thus the elementary thing in its wave state is in a state of potentiality. Since material particles appear with a specific mass in a specific point in space, when these particles revert to their wave state they leave the empirical world and exist again as a state of potentiality in the non-empirical universe. The implications are profound; this means instead of thinking of the empirical world as the primary reality, it is in fact the non-empirical cosmic background from which it emanates that is the primary reality, while the physical world is the secondary reality (Ponte & Schäfer, 2013). The nature of reality, quantum physics has shown, is that it is indivisible (Kafatos & Nadeau, 1990).

The wholeness of reality is further underscored by the following consideration: if the elementary things in their wave state of potentiality were not coherent, the empirical world that emanates from the wave of potentiality would be in a state of perpetual chaos. Yet it is not chaotic; the physical world appears to us as a logical and coherent system. As patterns of information, elementary things in their wave state of potentiality are a mental process (in other words not matter or real) and thoughts appear in the conscious mind; hence the concept of a conscious universe. In this conscious universe, our thinking is the realised potentiality of the cosmic mind which finds consciousness in us (Ponte & Schäfer, 2013). It is in this discovery of quantum physics that Jung's most seminal concept, the archetypical idea of the Unus Mundus developed with Marie-Louise von Franz finds vindication.

> Undoubtedly the idea of the Unus Mundus is founded on the assumption that the multiplicity of the empirical world rests on an underlying unity, and that not two or more fundamentally different worlds exist side by side or are mingled with one another. Rather, everything divided and different belongs to one and the same world, which is not the world of sense. (Jung, 1970, p. 767)

The Unus Mundus archetype implies that there is a reality that must be united, and that reality beyond the illusions of matter, division and opposites, is one. This is the concept that underlies the process of individuation which Robert Forman (1998) describes as the innate capacity of the individual to become aware of the self. The imperative of transformation is the impulse to unite what is divided.

Jung wrote that "I use the term 'individuation' to denote the process by which a person becomes a psychological 'individual,' that is, a separate, indivisible unity or 'whole'" (Jung, 1969, p. 275). The adherents of the Newtonian world of the material universe, consisting of matter and separate material things, were unable to accept Jung's propositions, and as a consequence, Jung's contribution was not well received

(Jaffé, 1989). Searching for wholeness in the material universe would be meaningless. But in the quantum world, Jung's contribution has found an empirical basis.

This search for wholeness is Jung's opus and is what underpins all of his work which found support in quantum physics where the meaning and purpose of humanity's existence is anchored in a unified, continuous reality. As Jung puts it:

> The main interest of my work is not concerned with the treatment of neurosis, but rather with the approach to the numinous. But the fact is that the approach to the numinous is the real therapy, and inasmuch as you attain to the numinous experience, you are released from the curse of pathology. Even the very disease takes on a numinous character. (Jaffé, 1989, p. 16)

From quantum physics to bioelectronics: Marion Wood's cellular theory of obesity in a Jungian context of the collective unconscious

As a natural extension of the idea of an interconnected universe, the central thesis of bioelectronics that living matter is able to process environmental cues and manifest these into physical form followed. Adamski puts it as follows: living matter has its own sense of conscious connectedness to the earth and it is through this connection that information transfers between the two. Consequently, living matter grows by storing electronic impulses from the earth's electromagnetic field in order to create what Adamski refers to as "permanent psychological structures" (2011, p. 568). Similarly, Fritz-Albert Popp and Lev Beloussov proposed in 2003 the phenomenon of "bio-photons emissions" which describes the ability of the photons on biological cells' DNA to release and transfer information between cells by means of electromagnetic waves in a range of frequencies. As a healthy physical body possesses more photons, it is better able to control luminescence, the strength of the electromagnetic signal as it were. The photons work in harmony with each other and operate on electromagnetic vibrations which continually transmit information to other photons and structures external to the biosystem in which they exist, making photons the "universal medium of information and electromagnetic processes" (Popp & Beloussov, 2003, p. 568). These processes affect the entire genetic code of an organism, including the electrical activity taking place in the human brain, and interlocks "light and the dynamic processes of life" (p. 568).

These interactions in the bioelectronics structure determine not only physical health or illness but also human behaviour. In addition, molecular biochemical reactions link the electronic processes in living matter with chemical systems to create living biosystems, and here is the link with quantum physics. Quantum theory suggests that all molecules in the cosmos are interconnected and that matter operates on two fundamentals: chemical and electric processes. Going further, quantum theory has shown that matter originates from waves existing in a state of potentiality in the cosmic mind, a state to which matter reverts when not interacted with; hence the empirical and non-empirical worlds are interconnected and the difference between them is less a matter of substance and more a matter of state.

Adamski sums it up in his conclusion:

> Bioelectric models show that the biological system not only saves information about the life of the individual in its ontogeny, but also saves lives in the process of generational dimension, which is connected to the phylo-genesis. This means that thanks to electronic properties, a biological system has various opportunities for recording information about the experiences of individuals, the environment in which they live, but also has the ability to transfer this information from generation to generation. (2011, p. 569)

The context created by the contribution of bioelectronics to quantum theory in how it relates to Jung's iteration of the collective unconscious led to the conclusion that information, in particular archetypical information, is transferred through the DNA of cells.

Jungian analysis: the cellular phenomenon of obesity

In her contribution to the obesity debate, Jungian analyst Marion Woodman explored the intra-cellular dynamics of the human body and concluded that the psychology of obesity translates into a cellular issue because cells, like molecules, are interconnected. She argued that, with the exception of the periods during which the quantum of cells increases, occurring in early childhood and puberty, the number of cells inside the human body remains constant, but their size increases.

People who suffered obesity in childhood tend to have up to three times more cells than those who maintained average body weight. The implication is therefore that when people with obesity lose weight, they never lose the fat cells although they can change the size of these cells as they become empty of the fat previously stored in them. However, nature abhors a vacuum; the cells demand to be replenished and do it by triggering the relapse cycle.

The cells send emergency signals to the brain to increase food consumption, overriding conscious willpower and the dieter succumbs. Food consumption increases and the cells return to their "normal state" at which point they become stable again. For Woodman, this hyper-cellularity is the driving force behind excessive food intake. As the fat cells rebel against the disturbance of the "homeostatic equilibrium", when these cells start emptying as a result of weight loss, it also overrides the human conscious willpower as it seeks to regain adiposity.

This is the process behind the onset of dieters' depression and highly variable mood states as they progress along their journey of weight loss. But as the complexes and psychic content of each individual differ, the manner in which the hyper-cellularity will manifest will similarly differ. Jung and Woodman, however, acknowledged that it would not be practical to develop an infinite series of highly customised weight loss and therapeutic interventions to individual requirements. Instead, the general point of departure is offered by the complexes—the contents of what Jung referred to as constellations.

Jung described constellations as external forces that are beyond one's control, but as she explains, the constellations steer one to take action when faced with an unacceptable situation. The active complexes trigger reactions to the forces emanating from the constellations, which in turn drives the active thinking required for the person to move to the transcendent function and embark on the hero's journey.

To test this thinking Woodman conducted Jung's word association tests on twenty women to gain insight into their complexes; the sample consisted of both obese and non-obese women. Her findings were that there were elements particularly prevalent in the obese group that did not exist at all or were of very low incidence in the normal weight group. These elements included a negative mother complex and negative animus, feelings of being caged in, aggression, and the tendency to eat for comfort in stressful situations in the obese women, echoing to some extent the findings of Freudian analyst, Hilde Bruch, in her observation that childhood obesity is associated with a lack of nurturing, particularly from the mother figure in early childhood (Bruch & Touraine, 1940).

Women with a high BMI do not only have different complexes than normal BMI women, high BMI women think very differently about food. Woodman found that obese women scored very high in the food category of the word association tests, while the others scored zero.

This finding emphasises high BMI women's obsession with food, as well as their tendency to use food as a method of self-punishment through starvation, as self-nurture when feeling emotionally vulnerable, and as scapegoat instead of acknowledging the feelings that sit behind overeating. Food, Woodman found, literally rules the existence, lives, and complexes of people with obesity. High BMI people indeed think very differently about food than normal BMI people, and this explains why people with obesity are far more sensitive to food cues than those of normal weight.

In addition, she found that people with obesity tend to vastly underestimate the grip that food has over their lives. Associated with that is the higher incidence of poor body image, fear of rejection, tendencies towards perfectionism, and hypersensitivity, revealed in the obese women's scores on the word association tests. Where the normal body weight and the obese women's scores did converge in the test scores, was around issues such as the presence of a negative father figure, an overweight father, the fear of taking responsibility for the consequences of personal actions, growing up to believe one was unwanted as a child, and having feelings of rejection as a result. While these complexes tend to overlap between the two groups, they seem to lie dormant in the unconscious insofar as weight is concerned, and therefore are not an influencing factor.

The inseparability between mind and body follows from the continuum between wave forms and matter established by the quantum physics discussion earlier in the chapter, and for the somatic dynamics of obesity to be understood, both mind and matter must be studied. Woodman concludes that regardless of any medical, nutritional, or physical solution proposed in the treatment of obesity, ultimately it is only the individual who can instinctively know how to deal with it by getting back in touch with the body and not regarding the body as the enemy, and by reintegrating the self by exploring and solving the complexes through the hero's journey of transformation.

Connecting the cells to the archetypes and the complexes

As mentioned earlier, a negative or complex and troublesome mother-son relationship tends to lead to a negative anima in the son and could translate into anything from oversensitivity and defensiveness to depression.

The Death Mother archetype is a "cold, fierce, violent and corrosive power" according to Daniela Sieff (2009, p. 178) and is a representation of the force of the negative anima. The Death Mother paints a dim picture of hopelessness and turmoil, and interprets the unknown in the grimmest of ways possible; this Death Mother prefers death over life as an outcome, and when faced with the Death Mother, trauma and destruction follow. The Death Mother's energy is drawn from the psyche; it originates in the self where she lies dormant, but the Death Mother energy can be triggered by someone close, often a person to whom one has dedicated faith and devotion (such as one's mother or life partner). Sieff illustrated the power of the Death Mother with reference to the initial rejection of a child by the mother which can be profound in its implications for the child. The child feels the mother no longer accepted him and this leads to overwhelming feelings of being rejected. This memory of rejection is then stored in the unconscious where it also becomes a fear of abandonment, not only bedevilling the person's relationships later in life but also translating into physical consequences such as cardiac arrhythmia and other physical symptoms which signal the presence of the Death Mother energy as it becomes part of one's physical cell structure and results in the body becoming self-destructive.

It is important to note that the energy of the Death Mother is self-generated and inflicted; she is "born out of despair ... incubated by the crushed hope of an unlived life ... the shadow side of disappointment ... and hopelessness" (Sieff, 2009, pp. 190–191), and only when acknowledging her presence in our life can we prevent the destruction of it.

When the Death Mother is present but not acknowledged, the unconscious in striving to regain balance in the psyche tends to develop defence mechanisms against the harsh lashings of the Death Mother. In the case of presenting as eating disorders, these defence mechanisms include "an armour of fat, oedema, vomiting; *anything* to keep the poison out" (Sieff, 2009, p. 179). Sieff noted that it is the Death Mother's energy within us that convinces us that we are not good enough or worthy enough of love and admiration, and this could in extreme cases translate into not allowing oneself to be loved or to experience love in any form. The Death Mother is cunning; she prohibits access to the other unconscious archetypes and thus the means to defeat her by limiting abstract and imaginative thinking through concretisation. By inhibiting the psyche's ability for imagination, she replaces the imaginative power of abstract thinking which allows the psyche to grasp the symbolic and metaphorical meanings emanating from the unconscious; the psyche's access to the unconscious is hindered. Once the symbolic and metaphorical content of the unconscious is interpreted literally, it loses its meaning; for example, unconscious content directed at producing growth along the ego/self axis interpreted literally by the psyche and the person becomes fat as they grow literally obese; but this growth is obviously destructive.

She explains further that the alcoholic, the drug addict, or in this instance, the overeater knows that they have to sacrifice the addictive substance if they want change in their lives, but the addiction is the coping mechanism they have established over the years to protect them from the Death Mother energy. To deal with it requires the hero's journey; for the person would have to unearth the trauma, access the unconscious by moving past the ego, and embark on the perilous journey of transformation resulting in individuation, for the Death Mother does not loosen her grip lightly. In some cases, the impulse for embarking on this journey of transformation requires that the person needs to be facing the final stage of their instilled illness, be it obesity, addiction, depression, or something else. For the threat of facing the physical death is sometimes the stimulus required to garner the strength of the Death Mother, and she warns that this journey is not for the fainthearted and that seeking guidance is imperative.

Sieff describes the process following the "turning point" in one's life as one in which the death energy is harnessed "in the service of life" (2009, p. 193), for the unknown is revealed and brought to consciousness as the rebirth takes place; the midwife being another archetype, the Apocalyptic Mother. It is during an apocalypse when everything which has been hidden from view is revealed as the Apocalyptic Mother engages the Death Mother in what Sieff describes as an epic struggle between life and death, for the Death Mother wants to destroy and "turns life into stone", but the Apocalyptic Mother "shatters the stone" (p. 194). This is the violent struggle of birth that walks parallel with the agonising pain of birth which is the necessary requirement for the personal transformation process needed to begin a new phase of life. The two archetypical Mothers are differentiated by their intentions; the Death Mother aims to destroy and kill so as to fulfil the ego's primitive urges while the Apocalyptic Mother's energy is imbedded in sacrifice and "the ego's surrender to the guidance of the self in order to transform destructive … into the creative flow of life" (pp. 194–195).

But the Apocalyptic Mother dispenses strong medicine; through her harsh penetration into the soul and breaking down the perceptions that derive from the concretised symbols the Death Mother favours (the ego), the patient finally regains access to the unconscious through which the true Self can be made whole as individuation is achieved.

The implication of the connected universe is that as we change, so the environment in which we find ourselves will also appear to be changing; note that we may discover that the situations or relationships in which we find ourselves no longer serve us as the transformative process progresses, and that during this time the advice is to remain open to the symbols that will keep rising from the unconscious while surrendering the ego's desire to resist change. She further noted that the Apocalyptic Mother is ever present, but that the choice to engage her remains that of the individual concerned; however, the choice is between the illusory comfort offered by the respectively destructive cycle of the Death Mother and the vastly disruptive, but ultimately freeing prospect offered by the Apocalyptic Mother. For, writes Sieff, "In the heart of death, I found the gift of life" (2009, p. 198).

Jung's second major archetype, the animus, represents the powers of reason, mental acuity, intelligence, and physical life, and is the masculine opposite of the intuitive, female anima, according to Aletheia Luna (2014). The animus energy derives from the father figure, and like the anima, when negative, can become "a demon of death" and operate in very similar ways to the Death Mother of the anima (Jung, von Franz, Henderson, Jacobi, & Jaffé, 1964, p. 199). While both sexes can suffer the impact of both the anima and the animus as both are present in males and females alike, it is often the negative animus, the Demon of Death that impacts women.

Luna explains further that the function of the animus when in its positive state is what drives the empowerment of people, in particular women, the development of confidence, and the quality of reason;

but when in its negative state, the animus energy is often manifested in aggressiveness, impulsivity, and insensitivity. Laura Martin (2016) observed that women mostly experience their animus as negative; a positive animus is quite rare among women. For her the animus and anima are contra-sexual images that are the most useful stepping stones in the transformation process towards individuation; they are embedded in the unconscious and are the "most opposite to the ego" (Martin, 2016, p. 30).

To illustrate her point, Martin cites the example of the female crime fiction writer Dorothy L. Sayers and how the character of her lead detective, Lord Peter Wimsey presents as the imaginary figure of Sayers's psyche and her conscious and unconscious experience of Wimsey as her animus. Sayers describes her Wimsey as a "largely unconscious figure that mediates between her conscious and unconscious, unlocking her creativity" (Martin, 2016, p. 28) and clearly illustrates Jung's concept of the syzygy. Wimsey is rich and casually indulges in the type of luxuries Sayers, at the time a struggling intellectual, could only dream of. She invented a character that was intellectual, witty, sensible, superior, and perfect in every sense of the word: all the qualities that she thought she did not have, and in so doing unconsciously attempted to restore balance by bestowing on her fictional character all the qualities she saw herself lacking.

The archetypes

Martin explains that Jung's archetypes are repetitive constructions of innate instincts that are used by the psyche to deal with physical life challenges (birth and death) and life role experiences (e.g. becoming a mother or father); these cannot be observed directly but must be interpreted through the perceptions of the person experiencing them. The archetypes offer the ego a degree of flexibility and operate inferior to, in contrast to, and external to the ego. It is in this that Jung's archetypes differ from those of Freud; for Freud saw the ego as stable and concrete and therefore unable to change. Jung's archetypes allow the ego to change through the individuation process.

For her the psyche goes out of balance when the female energy, the anima, in both men and women is suppressed. The unconscious battle that ensues can lead to physical disease and causes the persona—the "mask or outward face of the ego" (Martin, 2016, p. 31) to distort to the extent that the persona is no longer sustainable as an outward projection. The man who displays the outward persona of power and masculinity in the stereotypical sense and suppresses what he perceives as his weak side—the female energy of sensitivity and emotion, risks being overcome by it in the worst possible moment as the anima reacts to the persona.

Martin explains the difference between the complexes and the archetypes as follows: "An archetype may be said to constellate when it has a strongly felt significance to an individual or a group; in other words, when someone or some people have a complex related to the archetype" (2016, p. 33). Archetypes then exist in the collective unconscious and are experienced universally, but the manner in which they impact on the individual psyche depends on the individual's personal perception of the archetypes, and it is around the—perceptions that the complexes are developed.

Jung's iteration found some support among the cognitive school of psychology. Cognitive theorist Pyysiäinen describes a model in 2009 that is very similar to Jung's noting that:

> The architecture of the mind … shapes beliefs, thus creating cross-culturally recurrent patterns. This implies that not all concepts and beliefs have an equal potential for becoming widespread. The most successful representations in cultural selection are those that "match" people's mental architecture, in that an existing "slot" corresponds to the form of the representation in question. (Pyysiäinen, 2009, pp. 3–4)

According to Erik Goodwyn (2013), cognitive scientists agree with Jung's theory that there is a deeper meaning in cultural stories and it is linked to universal psychological functions, as the same golden thread of a story can be observed in many different cultures. However, the cognitive school stops short of accepting the archetypes. Goodwyn argues that these "universal commonalities in human cognition, emotion and memory" (2013, p. 395) that are typical of folk tales and legends endure as they are passed on from one person to the next, but that in the passing along, the stories evolve and change to reflect the cultural changes that may occur over time.

To evaluate these, Goodwyn proposed what he termed the "attractor state model" to enable the structured study of recurring motifs and how these relate to archetypes beyond mere theoretical speculation. The criteria of the model to be applied when evaluating folk tales and legends were that they had to be minimally counter-intuitive, rhythmic, and emotionally sharp narratives that deployed middle level objects and characters, and occur in an indistinct time and place setting. The plot had to be a simple conflict-oriented plot with dramatic reversals, and a sense of interconnectedness should be more resonant (that is, more memorable and "sticky") than a story without these qualities (2013, p. 403). He stated that through his model, one will be able to distinguish "more clearly which clinical narratives and dreams are more resonant [due to the] empirically derived set of criteria" (p. 404). He also advises that self-narratives of a client can have similarities to resonant narratives and through facilitated therapy, narratives can be explored in order to facilitate individuation.

Michael Faber and John Mayer described an archetype as "internal mental model of a typical, generic story character to which an observer might resonate emotionally" (2009, p. 307). According to them, archetypes often represent the main characters in narratives and hold conversant and repetitive traits that are related to life lessons or life stages. And Lindenfeld explained in 2009 that archetypes portray different facets of the personality, which is moulded by a person's environment and culture. He noted that archetypes are a symbolic manifestation of what represents a person's beliefs and disbeliefs, needs and doubts.

The hero's journey: an illustration of the hero archetype

To illustrate the relevance of the archetypal influence on an individual's everyday life, the example of the hero archetype and the concept of the Hero's Journey as explained by Joseph Campbell and David Kudler in 2004 will be discussed. Shadraconis associates the hero in his writings of 2013 with danger, trials and tribulations, nobility, strength, and triumph. The hero figure is conqueror of evil and the main storyline always illustrates the challenges the hero must overcome during his or her quest, while the ending is always "happily ever after" as the hero triumphs. As an archetype, the hero is the sense maker as it rationalises the events in a person's life, to understand what is happening and why.

As such, the hero re-establishes order in a chaotic psyche. The Hero's Journey is one of discovering knowledge and understanding, and as the process of transformation requires the sacrifice of the ego to achieve the wholeness of the self, individuation is not for the fainthearted; for the Hero's Journey requires not only sacrifice (of the ego) on the part of the hero, but also supernatural powers in metaphor. In some tales, the hero enthusiastically embarks on his journey, but in others, a reticent hero must be convinced by others or forced by circumstance to embark on the journey.

Campbell and Kudler described the hero's journey as consisting of different stages; the starting point finds the hero living a mundane everyday life, followed by the onset of the journey in the second phase triggered by an extreme situation or personal crisis. In modern fiction, this trigger point is often presented as an existential threat that is presented along the lines of the end of the world, or of America, but one man could save it … Stage three is where the hero recognises the challenge but is overwhelmed by the extent of the threat and, doubtful of his abilities to prevail, the hero initially is reluctant. But as the threat compounds and becomes ever more pressing, the hero becomes motivated to act. Stage four offers further inducements to action which in some tales are represented as the wise council of significant people in the hero's life who offer motivation and encouragement, or alternatively the appearance of a resource that would make the quest possible.

In stage five, the hero passes the contemplation stages and sets off in action and is now determined to embark on the adventurous journey into the unknown. Stage six sees the hero facing the trials and tribulations of his quest, but these serve to make him stronger so that when he reaches the most challenging part of his journey in stage seven, usually presented in the form of a test of courage, in that the hero has to pass through the underground cave where danger lurks, climb the mountain or otherwise pass through the Valley of the Shadow of Death, he is strong enough to complete the journey. It is on this part of the journey that the hero acquires his final piece of equipment or the insight he needs for the final battle, be it a magic sword or a ring. The perils of passage deepen in stage eight to the point where the hero is no longer certain of survival. The hero hits rock bottom at this stage and there is a significant change in the scene, usually the death or illness of a key ally or the loss of a critical resource that makes the passage possible.

Faced with such an amplified challenge set, the hero has to find new strength or have an epiphany that brings to light a new realisation, and a rebirth takes place. Emerging from stage eight, the hero enters stage nine stronger and wiser than ever before and ready to fight the final battle and prevails over his adversary; at this point in the story he gets the girl, but before he can set the captives free, be crowned king, and be triumphantly received in jubilation, which comes in stage eleven, the hero is not out of danger yet in stage ten; for having rescued the proverbial damsel in distress, the hero has to make his escape and in this is faced with the final, and often most vivid battle of the journey.

Stage eleven sees the hero emerging as a wiser and stronger person, for now the transformation is complete and is followed by the final stage in which the hero returns to his former mundane life as a changed person. While the circumstances and environment are as before, the hero appreciates his or her situation more and experiences it differently as a result of the wisdom and strength acquired on the journey.

The Hero's Journey is a metaphor illustrating the journey of transcendence and is quite evident in the Freudian and Jungian interpretations of Lewis Carroll's Alice texts, which will be discussed later in the book.

The obese hero's journey

As a hero is associated with danger, trials and tribulations, nobility, strength, and triumph (Shadraconis, 2013), the same associations can be made with a person on the journey of weight loss. The obese person continuously grapples with the limitless health dangers, as well as the health consequences of being obese (Mokdad et al., 2003). The trials and tribulations of the obese person's journey encapsulate the continuous mental struggle with issues such as poor body image, fear of rejection, tendencies towards perfectionism, and hypersensitivity. The hero figure is seen as the conqueror of evil and the main storyline always illustrates the challenges that the hero must overcome during his (or her) quest, while the ending is always "happily ever after" as the hero triumphs (Shadraconis, 2013).

In this instance the hero is the obese person, the conqueror of fat, bad eating habits, and negative self-talk, to mention a few of the challenges. As mentioned earlier, as an archetype, the hero is the sense maker as he or she rationalises the life events, to understand what is happening and why. As such, the hero re-establishes order in a chaotic psyche (Shadraconis, 2013). In the obese person's life, the subject needs to rationalise many situations, events, and feelings to understand why he or she is obese. Often these elements are stored as complexes in the unconscious and can be as deep-rooted as a negative mother complex and negative animus, which often surface as feelings of being caged in, aggression, or the tendency to eat for comfort in stressful situations, as explained by Marion Woodman. The Freudian analyst, Hilde Bruch, also spoke about childhood obesity that is associated with a lack of nurturing, particularly from the mother figure in early childhood (Bruch & Touraine, 1940).

To understand these issues and to discover the knowledge within, the Hero's Journey is inevitable. As a process of transformation, sacrifice of the ego is required to achieve the wholeness of the self. The Hero's Journey requires not only sacrifice (of the ego) on the part of the hero, but also supernatural powers in metaphor. In some tales, the hero enthusiastically embarks on his journey, but in others, a reticent hero must be convinced by others or forced by circumstances to embark on the journey. With the obese person, the quest often begins many times through life: New Year's resolutions, fitting into that pair of designer jeans, a friend who is following the ultimate diet programme and has lost five kilograms in just two weeks, doctor's orders to lose weight or else ... Regardless of the cause for action, the obese person decides to turn over a new leaf. Often enthusiastically or perhaps reluctantly, the obese person sets out on the journey of weight loss.

Twelve stages of the obese hero's journey towards successful weight loss

The starting point finds the hero living a mundane everyday life, followed by the onset of the journey. The obese person's life tends to be the same: for years an obese person lives day to day, consuming too many calories, not exercising enough, and ignoring the physical alarms of the body. In the second phase, a person is triggered by an extreme situation or personal crisis. Again, as mentioned earlier, a trigger can be anything from a negative physical test to an illness or it could be as insignificant as a negative comment. In modern fiction, this trigger point is often presented as an existential threat along the lines of the end of the world (usually America), but one man could save it ...

Stage three is where the hero recognises the challenge, but is over-whelmed by the extent of the threat and, doubtful of his or her abilities to prevail, the hero is initially reluctant. As the threat builds and becomes ever more pressing, the hero becomes motivated to act. Usually, the big-gest hurdle for the obese person, at this stage, is the reminiscence of often several failed attempts of weight loss. Again, many other internal as well as external factors can be included here: unsupportive family members, insufficient monetary funds to purchase healthy food, the daunting thought of a complete lifestyle change, etc. Stage four offers further inducements to action. In some tales, inducements are repre-sented as the wise counsel of significant people in the hero's life who offer motivation and encouragement, or alternatively the appearance of a resource that would make the quest possible. Motivation and encouragement from people surrounding the obese person can consist of anyone—from a concerned or caring friend or family member to a registered dietician. Usually, as in the typical hero's journey, the wise counsel of significant others comes from the many people in an obese person's immediate environment—not only physically, but in this mod-ern day and age, there is a whole new world of possible support that also exists in the virtual world of the internet.

In stage five, the hero passes the contemplation stages, sets off in action, and is now determined to embark on the adventurous journey into the unknown. At this stage, the obese person has made that deci-sion to set out on the road to weight loss. Usually during this stage, a diet plan will be established, perhaps also an exercise plan that prom-ises optimal results. The plan of action will vary from person to person. Some people will prefer to follow a diet or exercise plan that someone they know had used to achieve promising results, some may consult a registered dietician or a biokineticist, some people may decide to follow a holistic route and consult a spiritualist of some sort. Regardless of the path taken, the obese person believes that the chosen plan of action is the golden ticket to success.

Stage six sees the hero facing the trials and tribulations of his or her quest, but these serve to make him or her stronger. The obese per-son is faced daily with temptations: the smell of freshly baked bread in the local grocery store, an office birthday celebration with "just one small piece of cake", hunger pains that are more prevalent in the obese person's imagination than is realistically possible ... When he or she reaches the most challenging part of the journey in stage seven, usually presented in the form of a test of courage, in that the hero has to pass through the underground cave where danger lurks, climb the mountain or otherwise pass through the Valley of the Shadow of Death, he or she is by now strong enough to complete the journey. It is on this part of the journey that the hero acquires the final piece of equipment or insight he or she needs for the final battle, be it a magical sword or a ring. At this stage, the obese person has been able to stick to the plan for a while or for a few days. From nowhere, an incredible sense of hunger, an overwhelming need for any kind of food that is not healthy, creeps into the obese person's existence like a destroying monster. All the obese person can think of is failing … Eating … giving up on the chosen path. The perils of passage deepen in stage eight to the point where the hero is no longer certain of survival.

The hero hits rock bottom at this stage and there is a significant change in the scene, usually the death or illness of a key ally or the loss of a critical resource that makes the passage possible. This stage has been scientifically explained by Marion Woodman in the intracellular dynamics of the human body, as mentioned earlier. She concluded that the psychology of obesity translates into a cellular issue when the fat cells demand to be replenished and does it by triggering the relapse cycle. The solution for this stage lies in her conclusion: that regardless of any medical, nutritional, or physical solution proposed in the treatment of obesity, ultimately it is only the individual who can instinctively know how to deal with it by getting back in touch with the body and not regarding the body as the enemy, and by reintegrating the self by exploring and solving the complexes through the hero's journey of transformation.

Faced with such an amplified set of challenges, the hero has to find new strength or have an epiphany that brings to light a new realisation, and causes a rebirth to take place. Emerging from stage eight, the hero enters stage nine stronger and wiser than ever before and ready to fight the final battle, prevailing over the adversary, in this case, obesity. By resisting the soul-slaying temptations, by coaxing oneself through the darkness of the self-destruction of obesity, and having discovered unknown strength within, the obese person continues on this Hero's Journey. It is at this stage that many people fail in their weight loss aims. The temptation becomes too overwhelming, the darkness of self-destruction sets in, and the undiscovered strength remains hidden under the unresolved issues of the unconscious.

In stage ten, the hero is not out of danger yet; for having rescued the proverbial damsel in distress, the hero has to make his escape and in this is faced with the final, and often most vivid battle of the journey. Just as the obese person has found renewed strength and will to carry on with a reformed lifestyle, he or she is faced with a fork in the road. The obese person is once again confronted with the same demons as before, but in order to address the issue not only on the surface, to prevent the same obstacles from repeating themselves over and over again, the obese person has to solve the underlying issue. In other words, instead of dealing with the cravings, the hunger, or the need for comfort food, the obese person has to find the connection in the unconscious. The existing complex in the unconscious must be acknowledged and resolved in order to be solved and for transformation to take place.

Stage eleven sees the hero emerging as a wiser and stronger person, for now the transformation is complete and is followed by the final stage in which the hero returns to his former mundane life as a changed person. While the circumstances and environment is as before, the hero appreciates his or her situation more and experiences it differently as a result of the wisdom and strength acquired on the journey. After resolving the issues that feed obesity in an individual, the person now knows how to cope with the daily challenges that he or she faces during the weight loss journey. Triggers can now be recognised and understood at a deeper level and therefore better resolved.

The full circle

In many cases, the obese person completes the full circle of the Hero's Journey by reaching ideal weight, but gradually regains the weight. This is an indication that all issues in the unconscious have not been resolved and the journey of transformation is incomplete.

The Hero's Journey will commence once again, often with more weight and health issues than the previous one. With every attempt, embarking on the Hero's Journey becomes increasingly difficult, as the success of the previous attempt is contrasted with the failure to sustain a healthy lifestyle. However, the denial of pressing underlying issues becomes more difficult every time, which forces the obese person back onto the Hero's Journey.

The Hero's Journey is a metaphor illustrating the journey of transcendence. It is quite evident that the successful journey of the obese person is no easy task, just as change is no easy task for any person.

In order to achieve successful and sustained weight loss, the obese person has to undergo his own Hero's Journey towards individuation; not only by following a healthy eating plan and doing regular exercise, but also by addressing all the disparaging issues that are suppressed in the unconscious.

Jungian reading of the Alice text: going into the rabbit hole and *Through the Looking Glass*—a tale of a young woman's journey into the personal unconscious

To illustrate the importance of the Hero's Journey and the significant role that the unconscious symbols play in the conscious behaviour of the obese person, Lewis Carroll's book on the adventures of *Alice in Wonderland*, and its follow-up *Through the Looking Glass*, can serve as a classic example. In these two books we see that the development of Alice has two phases; the first—as depicted in *Alice in Wonderland* is a coming-of-age tale, while in the later *Through the Looking Glass*, Alice returns as an adult facing a life crisis in the Victorian version of the Hero's Journey. The following analysis illustrates just how convoluted symbols and complexes from the unconscious could be and how conscious thoughts and behaviour can become so chaotic and utterly confusing in a sense, due to these influences from the unconscious.

Lewis Carroll's tale, *Alice in Wonderland*, starts off with a nightmare about following a white rabbit and falling into a dark hole. From a Jungian perspective, the image and story of the rabbit hole is the starting point for Alice's journey into her unconscious, featuring perils to overcome and animal guides representing different aspects of her unconscious providing insights along the way. As she progresses on her journey, Alice experiences the increase in consciousness which is at the core of the individuation process described by Jung as required for the development of the individual personality (Edinger, 1963 as cited in Elder & Cordic, 2009). When she arrives at the other end of the rabbit hole, Alice enters Wonderland—a place of strange logic and exotic creatures featuring a dodo bird, the white rabbit, the Cheshire cat, and a blue caterpillar, a Mad Hatter and a Queen of Hearts. Upon waking up, she shares the nightmare with her father and expresses her fear that she may have gone mad, upon which her father replies that all the best people are mad, illustrating Joseph Campbell's (2002) reluctant hero uncertain of whether to make the journey.

Alice starts her journey betrothed to a young man of "good stock" whom it would be very sensible to marry, and finds herself faced with a life decision of enormous consequence; for the decision to marry Hamish or not will impact the rest of her life. At this point, Alice notices the white rabbit who she intuits she must follow. Her journey into Wonderland starts with a fall—illustrative of the archetypical fall which precedes the journey into the unconscious (Goldschmidt, 1933).

At the beginning of the journey, Alice is confused—she is unsure whether this great adventure is real or whether she has not plainly lost her mind. In her attempt to make sense of Wonderland she questions everything, but gets frustrated by the twisted logic of Wonderland at every turn. One of the key themes that emerges in Wonderland (the unconscious) is that it appears to the conscious mind as a meaningless puzzle—Alice encounters a series of puzzles that seem to have no solutions, imitating the manner in which life tends to frustrate expectations (Greenacre, 1955). Alice expects that her encounters with the characters in Wonderland will help her make meaning and sense of it, but is frustrated at every turn, from attempting to solve the Mad Hatter's riddle, to the Caucus race, failing to understand the Red Queen's croquet game—and in each instance the riddles and challenges presented to Alice in Wonderland appear to have no purpose or have no logical answer. This describes how unfathomable the unconscious is to the logical approach of the conscious (Goldschmidt, 1933). Alice soon learns that the riddles of Wonderland cannot be solved by reason or logic, and in this Carroll illustrates how the unconscious frustrates rational expectations and resists logical interpretation, even when the content seems familiar or the challenges solvable on the surface (Goldschmidt, 1933).

All the creatures of the story are waiting for *the* Alice (the individuated *Self* that emerges after transformation) as it was prophesied that *the* Alice will slay the dragon that is oppressing all in Wonderland and in the process, reclaim the land for the White Queen. The only problem is that they are not sure whether this Alice is "the right Alice" or the "wrong Alice"—for to overcome the dragon, Alice has to be the right Alice. Wonderland (the unconscious) is a place where danger lurks, and as Edinger noted, Jung was fond of quoting Holderlin who said where danger is, grows also the rescuing power.

Upon arriving in Wonderland, Alice thinks that it is she (her ego) that consciously directs her path in life, but in the story, she befriends a dog (often represented in dreams as instinct). The dog gives her a warning not to diverge from the path, to which Alice—in the ego state she is naïve insofar as the operations of the unconscious are concerned—replies that she makes her own path. She speaks as if she is truly convinced that it is in her best interests to allow the "rational" ego to direct her path, which is exactly what the dog (her instinct), warns her not to do, for to survive in Wonderland, rationality won't serve Alice (Greenacre, 1955).

Another aspect of Alice's unconscious manifests as the blue cater-pillar (the symbol of transformation) who says to her "you are almost Alice". At this stage Alice is more receptive to the caterpillar, as she has learned by this point in the story that it is not the ego that creates the path, and as such she understands that the animals—representing the different aspects of her unconscious, can be trusted to serve as guides. As she progresses on her journey into the unconscious, the aberrant logic of the creatures in Wonderland that so irritated her in the beginning when she was still trying to assert her ego, starts making sense to Alice as she sees that the irrational, "mad" creatures actually have much to offer her on her journey towards greater consciousness, as explained by Phyllis Greenacre in 1955. This is seen in Alice's encounter with the Cheshire cat who, like the other creatures, uses the irrational logic of Wonderland— to prove that he is mad by drawing flawed conclusions from faulty assumptions. When Alice confronts him, he changes the subject, leaving her frustrated.

> "And how do you know that you're mad?"
>> "To begin with," said the Cat, "a dog's not mad. You grant that?"
>> "I suppose so," said Alice.
>> "Well, then," the Cat went on, "you see a dog growls when it's angry, and wags its tail when it's pleased. Now I growl when I'm pleased, and wag my tail when I'm angry. Therefore, I'm mad. (Carroll, 2008, p. 65)

The Cheshire cat maintains calm, grinning outsider status throughout. He reveals to Alice an insight into the workings of Wonderland that did not occur to her. First, Wonderland as a place (the unconscious) is indeed mad and has a stronger cumulative effect than any of its citizens (the creatures, symbolising different aspects of Alice's uncon-scious). Because Wonderland is ruled by nonsense, Alice's rationality is inconsistent with Wonderland's operating principles and therefore she becomes frustrated, and the other creatures in Wonderland experience Alice as mad and rude in turn. But, reveals the Cheshire cat, if Alice had to embrace the madness of Wonderland, she would understand it and the creatures would engage her.

In Jungian terms, the Cheshire cat acts as guide to Alice and it is through him that we learn that the unconscious is not rational, and cannot be accessed through the reason of the conscious but rather through the symbolism (Jung, 1959, 1963). It is the cat that leads Alice to the March Hare's house—the scene of the mad tea party—and later he leads her to the garden, her final destination. The cat seems to have privileged knowledge of Wonderland, and combined with his ability to manifest and disappear at will—in disembodied form, the cat also represents an element of the supernatural (Edinger cited in Elder & Cordic, 2009). Later the cat appears again, this time on the Queen of Hearts's croquet court, and Alice is quite pleased to see him again.

> *"How are you getting on?" said the Cat, as soon as there was mouth enough for it to speak with ... Alice put down her flamingo, and began an account of the game, feeling very glad she had someone to listen to her ...* (Carroll, 2008, p. 80)

In contrast, the Queen of Hearts (Death Mother) is not as concerned with nonsense and the perversions of logic that characterise life in Wonderland, but this is the character Alice must face to figure out the puzzle of Wonderland (Edinger, 1999 as cited in Elder & Cordic, 2009). She is literally at the heart of Alice's conflict, for this is the ruler who usurped Wonderland and that Alice must depose so that the land— now withered and out of balance, can be restored to the White Queen. The Queen of Hearts as a symbol of Alice's Death Mother archetype is obsessed with absolute rule and execution; she is a singular source of fear who dominates even the King of Hearts (Goldschmidt, 1933).

Even though Alice understands that the Queen of Hearts is merely a playing card (deriving from her own psyche), and after the Gryphon assured her that although the Queen regularly yells "off with their heads" nobody actually gets executed, and that the Queen's power lies in her rhetoric, to face her, Alice has to face her true fear of the Queen (Edinger, 1999 as cited in Elder & Cordic, 2009). It is the Queen's dismissive attitude to Wonderland that leads to the impression that Wonderland (the unconscious) is without substance, as it is devoid of logic. And to overcome this lack of logic, Alice repeatedly returns to analysis as seen in her approach to the chess game—her aim is to become sovereign, a queen rather than a pawn, and to do so she seeks to make meanings and test them against common reality (Edinger, 1999 as cited in Elder & Cordic, 2009).

> *"I'm sure I didn't mean …"* Alice was beginning, but the Red Queen interrupted impatiently.
>
> *"That's just what I complain of! You should have meant! What do you suppose is the use of a child without any meaning? Even a joke should have some meaning and a child is much more important than a joke, I hope. You couldn't deny that, even if you tried with both hands."*
> (Carroll, 2008, p. 217)

Megan Lloyd, as cited by William Irwin and Richard Brian Davis in 2009, describes Alice as the "unruly Alice", quite the departure from the pliable Cinderella and the passive Snow White who required male aid to bring them to life and consciousness again. Alice is the courageous heroine who was prepared to go into the unknown, not knowing whether she would emerge again and Lloyd reminds us that Alice, in doing so, rejected the stereotypical female submissive role. Just prior to the closing scene of the Walt Disney version of *Alice in Wonderland*, in which Alice takes up her sword to fight the dragon with the help of her creature friends, she finds the blue caterpillar who is turning into a cocoon, and laments, "You are going to die," to which the caterpillar replies, "No, I am going to be transformed." In this, Alice projects onto the caterpillar and illustrates the Jungian concept of synchronicity, as in seeing his change she immediately fears her own death as the likely outcome of her fight with the dragon, as her inner psychological process is reflected—like the caterpillar, Alice's own transformation will be achieved by overcoming the dragon, but to achieve it, she must face the risk of death (Woolverton & Burton, 2010).

The transcendence occurs for Alice as she overcomes the mighty dragon that is the champion of the Queen of Hearts (Death Mother) and restores Wonderland to the White Queen. She found a source of power she did not know she had and she used this power for the greater good. Order is restored in the land (balance achieved again in the psyche) and the White Queen rules again, and Alice proves to herself and the other inhabitants of Wonderland that she is in fact the right Alice—she became herself as the individuation is achieved (Jung, 1963). Having done so, Alice knows that she must leave her unconscious Wonderland as she has found her purpose and now there "are questions I must answer, things I have to do". Alice climbs out of the rabbit hole to return "home" and finds her intended groom waiting for her where she left him, and pronounces simply and boldly to the astonished Hamish that she will not marry him as he is not the right man for her.

Alice entered Wonderland as a confused child and exited it as a woman; a woman who has found the inner courage to cast aside societal expectations—not as a trite act of meaningless rebellion, but as she was called to something greater. The story ends with Alice on the deck of the ship where she has been accepted as an apprentice. At the beginning of the story a large part of the pressure on Alice to marry Hamish was that Hamish was wealthy and would provide for Alice; after the transformation in Wonderland, Alice is able to provide for herself and therefore no longer needs to marry Hamish. At this point the blue butterfly lands on her shoulder. Alice recognises it as her friend, the transformed caterpillar and realises her own transformation is validated by the appearance of this symbol, according to Edinger (1999 as cited in Elder & Cordic, 2009). By answering the call and following the white rabbit into the unknown, Alice transformed from a dependent child who needed to secure her future through marriage to one who has embraced a path of wholeness and a personal meaning that cannot be found simply by trying to fit into others' expectations at the cost of the true self (Irwin & Davis, 2009).

Central to Jung's psychology is the achievement of individuation which requires the discovery of unconscious content to make this conscious so that we can become what we are at the essence of our being. Individuation is achieved by exploring the interplay between and transcending the opposites (Jung, 1959, 1963). This process is poignantly illustrated in *Alice in Wonderland* as she faces the Jabberwocky—the Red Queen's dragon. The Jabberwocky, when seeing Alice, says that it is a long time since they have done battle and that it was good to see her on the battlefield again; to which Alice replied that it was the first time she had met the Jabberwocky. The Jabberwocky replied that it is not Alice he was addressing, but the vorpal sword that he was speaking to, as depicted in the Disney movie *Alice in Wonderland* of 2010. The sword Alice was carrying, according to Absalom the blue caterpillar, knew what it needed to do. In preparing her for the battle the caterpillar cautions Alice to let the sword do what it wants to as it knows what it is doing and will defeat the

Jabberwocky. In this instance, in facing the demons of the unconscious (the Jabberwocky), the insignificant sword bearer is the conscious, who needs to let the far more powerful and knowing unconscious do what it must to defeat and overcome what ails the psyche.

Jung and gender

Susan Rowland points out that "A defining feature of Jung's treatment of gender is his placing of the feminine at the centre of his psychology while at the same time displacing women as social, material and historical beings" (2002, p. 44). Although, as Rowland's work illustrates, masculine bias in Jungian thinking can be mitigated by a more deconstructive reading, nevertheless Jungian psychology often appears to fit women with what we might call the anima's glass slipper. Some of Jung's pronouncements, when taken at face value, seem to suggest that women's "consciousness is characterised more by the connective quality of Eros and who are by definition a more primitive, relational, and instinctual being". In women, Jung states in his essay on anima and animus, "Eros is an expression of their true nature, while their Logos is often only a regrettable accident" (Jung, 1982, p. 171). In the tale of the twelve dancing princesses (Grimm & Grimm, 1884), the feminist contribution to Jungian interpretation sought to revise and extend these limiting assumptions. Little Grace emerges in this interpretation of the tale as an individuating force to embody the story's transformative consciousness, and she must differentiate herself from her sisters and emerge from her immersion in the collective anima. The subterranean world the princesses enter every night can be seen as a dream from which they find it impossible to wake. The King (ego, consciousness) has, in effect, buried them alive. But it is the combined force of their own addictive pleasures (the compulsive repetitive patterns Freud spoke of) and their collective insistence on conformity that makes it impossible to consider escape (the Death Mother archetype). Thus, unless subjected to outside intervention (the crisis of the psyche), they are doomed to move back and forth between morning and night, between upper- and underworlds in an endlessly repetitive cycle of descent and return, without ever being able to reap their journey's potential rewards. But it is possible to escape from the subterranean world for it has another side in which hidden things can be nurtured until they reach the light of day (the Apocalyptic Mother).

The book Little Grace has secured under her mattress is such a secret thing, the first of several hidden stories whose collective power will eventually combat the King's dominant narrative. Little Grace signals a growing resistance to her sisters "imprisonment in unthinking conformity". Though she too dances in the subterranean depths, the feminine does not simply happen to her as a kind of fate. Instead, she has begun to read her woman's life, a skill that allows her a separate psychic space where she can trust, and follow, her own intuitions. Her skill also permits her to look beyond personal concerns to read the signs of the culture. In these readings, she has the added support of the trees of silver, gold, and diamonds. The World Tree, frequently associated with the mother archetype, often appears in goddess-centred stories as a source of abundance, its fruit offered generously to any human supplicant, as depicted by Joseph Campbell in 1968. The fruit produced by the trees in the underworld provide a valuable light, by means of which Little Grace is able to foresee the individuation process beckoning just ahead.

The transition to Jungian feminism introduces the realm of the matriarchate, specifically that of the mythical figure known as the Kore, explained by Erich Neumann in 1955, who finds expression in the Demeter/Persephone story where the Kore figure, after descending to the underworld, experiences a subsequent rebirth. Persephone, as the seed that has been buried in the earth for the winter months, comes to life again in the spring; she has been initiated, through her sufferings, into the mysteries of transformation.

Jungian feminism further defines the transformative process as it occurs for women by suggesting that the shadow should be taken as a cultural as well as a personal phenomenon. Irene De Castillejo (1973) includes, as a necessary part of female individuation, the task of making conscious the shadow elements that have collected around women as participants in patriarchy. The collective female shadow first materialised when various god-centred nomadic tribes began to conquer and control settled goddess-centred communities around 2500 BCE. Eventually, the mother/daughter configuration that had originally characterised the Great Mother became split into distinct entities. Aspects of the Great Mother were differentiated into individualised figures and subsumed under patriarchy as the wives and daughters of the father gods; the mother aspect, as a representative of the old chthonic order, was forgotten or relegated to the underworld. Here she took up residence as Hecate,

Medusa, or Ereshkigal, powerful female figures associated with the earth, with darkness and, in some cases, with evil (Wolkstein & Kramer, 1983).

This mythological development has its psychological counter-part. The archetype of the Great Mother carries a negative underside. This dark aspect of the mother has found its way into masculine mythology and psychology as the female dragon, the Stone Mother, the castrating terror, whose powers must be destroyed once and for all to enable the male hero to attain maturity. From a female perspective, the witch can now be seen as a cultural shadow-construction that embodies male fears of female power (the vagina dentata). Instead of either destroying or disavowing this shadow, however, Jungian feminism suggests that it be brought to consciousness where its energies can be affirmed and utilised (Woolf, 1957).

Thus, in the story of the dancing princesses, instead of running away from what she has been taught to despise, Little Grace stands her ground. An enormous challenge faces her: to see these women not as a monolithic evil presence but as interesting and powerful aspects of herself. To break the spell, this is the mirror she must confront, accept, and eventually step through. What has been disguised by the dominant patriarchal narrative as ugly, dangerous, and life destroying, becomes something else as Little Grace faces the looking glass. Suddenly feminine self-assertion, including all those parts of the self which are considered unacceptable by conventional culture, is no longer something that must be hidden away, repressed, or denied. Instead, it can now be seen as a source of personal power that allows body and spirit to inhabit the world freely, without shame or apology. The looking glass stands as a door between two worlds. On one side is the timeless realm of fairy tale, characterised by unreflective repetition, in which women are expected to adhere to narrowly defined domestic roles. On the other side is a world marked by time and history in which strong women are increasingly able to act as self-defining agents of change.

Unfortunately, the tale does not end with a simplistic, one-dimensional happily ever after. The castle Grace returns to is in disarray and she resists enclosure within marriage (conjunctions), offered by Jungian theory as the goal of individuation, and thus, construction of the integrated self is not achieved. Yet, this "failure" is consistent with the deconstructive insight that such a union with the unconscious is impossible to maintain beyond brief moments (Rowland, 2002).

CHAPTER 7

Concept five: the personal unconscious (the Freudian perspective)

F reud's focus was on the individual. He believed that all issues manifested within the individual. When the story of Alice is analysed in this section, it becomes evident that Freud looked at Alice as the dream of the author, Lewis Carroll. Thus Alice is not analysed as the character in her own right (as in the Jungian discussion of Alice) but rather as a dream of the author and what it tells us about the author. The Freudian perspective will be discussed briefly, as it has been extensively discussed and compared throughout the previous concepts.

In brief, Freud proposed a psychoanalytic framework that identified the three forces of the psyche as the id, ego, and superego.

The id is unconscious and comprises everything that was present in the human psyche at birth, everything that is inherited and the instincts. The ego, being the conscious that fulfils the role of internal moderator between the animal instincts of the id and the social context of the external world, it is the link between the id and the external world and is aware of the stimuli that world presents. The ego responds to these stimuli by adapting to the external world in a manner that would maximise pleasure and avoid displeasure.

The superego represents the influence of authority figures including parents, teachers, and role models and also embodies their cultural values, customs, and behaviours; its function is to constrain satisfactions sought by the id and ego within the cultural context of external authority. Freud argued that the instincts originating in the id are the driving forces of all behaviour and identified them as Eros (love) and the destructive or death instinct; the purpose of the love instinct is to form connections and to preserve unity through its relationships with others. In contrast the death instinct seeks to undo connections and unity through destruction. Freud further posited that these two instincts can operate either exclusively from each other, or combine through attraction (Freud, 1940a, p. 190).

Freud's view of the human psychological process distinguishes between the conscious, preconscious, and unconscious (1940a, p. 31). In the conscious domain one is aware of ideas, but only briefly, while preconscious ideas are ideas that are capable of becoming conscious, but are not yet conscious. Unconscious ideas are not easily accessible, but they can be inferred, recognised, and explained through analysis (p. 32). Freud held that the unconscious thoughts of the id attempted to force their way into consciousness through dreams which can originate either in the id or the ego. The dreams are characterised by their strong use of symbolism and are the product of conflict and have the power to either bring up memories the dreamer had forgotten or to bring up impressions which cannot have originated from the dreamer's mind—and Freud cautioned that what the individual recalls from the dream is only the façade behind which the meaning must be inferred (p. 45).

Freud noted that the suppression of unconscious thoughts, emotions, and memories is the defence mechanism the ego deploys to protect itself from the real emotions and inner conflict that these events may produce.

The contribution of Freud to the subsequent development of analytical psychology

By presenting the concept of the collective unconscious, Jung's departure from the basis of psychology created by Freud is most clearly seen. Freud argued for the personal unconscious as a place where unresolved trauma hides, but made no provision for an interconnected, collective consciousness. The Freudian archetypes are metaphors describing recurring patterns in the individual; not the archetypes of Jung which tend more to describe an underlying cosmic reality.

Where Freud enabled Jung's contribution is in recognising the existence of the unconscious and providing one of the early descriptions of its functioning, including the apparent irrationality of the unconscious and its modality of symbols, as well as the introduction of the first archetypes. Jung took these ideas much further, but as the Freudian vs. Jungian interpretations of the Alice texts show in the discussion, instead of reading Freud and Jung as differing and separate theories, they should be read together as a continuum for there is value in both.

For Freud, the journey to wholeness is about reintegrating the broken pieces of a scattered psyche into a whole self, one which is in balance, and one in which the unconscious has been made conscious. The implication that follows is that once the underlying trauma feeding the behavioural pathology is resolved and made whole, the pathological behaviour, deprived of the trauma that feeds it, will no longer sustain itself. Thus, the obese person who overeats in response to trauma will no longer need to do so in compensation for a damaged psyche; for the pathological behaviour is an attempt to restore balance to a psyche that is out of balance. If this is the case, then obesity is the physical manifestation of a pathological behaviour pattern generated in the unconscious as a coping mechanism to compensate for and deal with the underlying trauma.

Jung similarly held the view that the psyche has a natural and innate urge towards wholeness, but goes further in introducing the concept of transcendence, as Joseph Henderson writes:

> A sense of completeness is achieved through a union of the consciousness with the unconscious contents of the mind. Out of this union arises what Jung called "the transcendent function of the psyche", by which a man can achieve his highest goal: the full realisation of the potential of his individual Self. (Jung, von Franz, Henderson, Jacobi, & Jaffé, 1964, p. 146)

Jung was fascinated by alchemy and specifically with the Philosopher's Stone which he saw as a metaphor for the process of individuation, the transformational journey into the wholeness in which the invisible is brought into the visible, matter is spiritualised, and where the spiritual becomes materialised; for Jung's wholeness derives from a personal and a collective unconscious, yet his consciousness achieved through individuation is decidedly personal. This path, however, requires the existence of a non-empirical domain of reality which Jung referred to as the collective unconscious. It is the collective unconscious which provides the infinite field for the progress of the ego-self axis relation. It is also the collective unconscious which nurtures the development of consciousness as the phenomena of the personal unconscious collapse (for example the transformation of the archetype of the Death Mother into the Apocalyptic Mother).

Differences between Freud and Jung

The difference between Jung's analytical psychology and Freud's psychoanalysis is evident in Jung's assumptions which reflect his theoretical differences with Freud. Jung agreed with Freud on the influences of childhood and past experiences on later behaviour, but unlike Freud, posited that behaviour is also shaped by future aspirations (Jung, 1948). Where Freud limited the libido to sexual energy, Jung saw it as a generalised psychic energy, but like Freud, Jung saw the psyche as being made up of a number of separate but interacting systems. For Jung, these systems were the ego, the personal unconscious, and went further than Freud in introducing the concept of the collective unconscious (Jung, 1948).

Jung saw the ego as representing the conscious mind and as being largely responsible for identity and continuity, and like Freud, Jung (1961) emphasised the importance of the conscious in the forming of personality, but departed from Freud in proposing that the unconscious consisted of two layers which he defined as the personal unconscious (similar to Freud's version of the unconscious), and the collective or transparent unconscious as the second layer. Jung also added the feature of complexes to the personal unconscious which he defined as a collection of thoughts, feelings, attitudes, and memories that form a single concept.

The influence of the complex on the individual increases as more elements attach to the complex, and Jung argued that the personal unconscious was much nearer to the surface (conscious) than Freud suggested.

By far the most notable difference between Freud and Jung was Jung's introduction of the collective or transpersonal unconscious which he saw as a level of unconscious shared collectively with other humans and which comprises latent memories of our evolutionary, cultural, and historical (or ancestral) past, and concluded that "the form of the world into which a person is born is already inborn in him as a virtual image" (Jung, 1953, p. 188). Jung referred to these ancestral images as archetypes which are images and thoughts that have universal meanings across cultures. Archetypes are expressed in dreams, literature, art, and religion and Jung explained that the reason why some symbols have the same meaning across different cultures was because they derive from archetypes shared by the whole of humanity. Hence, Jung believed that the basis for human behaviour lies in our primitive past which directs the human psyche.

The Freudian reading of the Alice texts

To illustrate the phenomenal differences between Jungian and Freudian interpretations, the Alice texts will be used as an example again. The psychoanalytic interpretation of *Alice in Wonderland* starts from the Freudian premise that the unconscious self is the repository of painful experience and repressed emotions and that our daily lives are spent moderating between the impulses and demands of the id, ego, and superego, according to William Empson in 1935. The psychoanalytic school of literary criticism holds that one can better appreciate literary works by applying the techniques of Freudian psychoanalysis to both literary characters and their authors, and to do so the literary work is treated as a dream in which the hidden meaning is found by means of a detailed analysis of both the language and symbolism featured in the literary work. In the case of *Alice*, the story begs for psychoanalysis because it is a dream. According to Empson, "To make the dream story from which *Alice in Wonderland* was elaborated seem Freudian, one only has to tell it" (1935, p. 357).

Unsurprisingly the first wave of Freudian analysis applied to Alice focused on the sexual symbolism, which according to Freudian theory reveals the repressed sexuality of the author, Lewis Carroll (Goldschmidt, 1933). Anthony Goldschmidt interprets Alice's ordeal in the hallway of doors as follows:

> ... the common symbolism of lock and key representing coitus, while the doors of normal size represent adult women which are disregarded by the author whose interest is centred on the little door which clearly symbolises little girls while the curtain in front

of the little door represent the female child's clothes, thus revealing
an undertone of paedophilia on the part of the author. (1933, p. 281)

From this perspective, Alice becomes a study in repressed male sexuality that Goldschmidt describes as an "unmarried clergyman of the
strictest virtue with a well-documented penchant for making child-
friends" and noted that it "does not require a great interpretative leap"
to believe that such a man might unconsciously relive this tension
through his writing (p. 281). For the Freudians, Alice provides a highly
sexualised reading. Goldschmidt noted events such as Alice's "pene-
trating" the rabbit hole, the keys and the locks and the small door as
colourful symbols of sexual intercourse which he interprets as proof of
the "presence in [Lewis Carroll's] subconscious of an abnormal emotion
of considerable strength" (p. 281). Goldschmidt's sentiments are echoed
by Schilder in 1971, who interprets the extreme violence of Wonderland
and its creatures as a representation of Carroll's frustrated sexual urges
and noted that his fascination with Alice reveals the complexities of his
frustrated sexual urges, for Alice was not only his love interest but also
acts as a substitute for mother and sister, thus revealing his repressed
desire to reject his adult masculinity and to become a little girl (Schilder,
1971, p. 291). Alice was in fact Alice Liddell, Lewis Carroll's favourite
among the daughters of his friends and thought to be the person for
whom he wrote the stories.

Later Freudian analysis focused more on the child and her identity
in interpreting Alice's experiences in Wonderland as an allegory for the
developing ego as the child mind learns how to understand the world
and the self. Stowell noted in 1983 that like all children, Alice must
separate herself from identification with others, develop an ego, and
become aware of her own and others' aggression, and learn to toler-
ate adversity without succumbing to self-pity. In other words, Alice has
to grow up. Identification is a recurring theme in *Alice in Wonderland*,
where the creatures constantly ask her to identify herself, but often she
finds herself unable to do so.

"Who are you?" said the caterpillar.

This was not an encouraging opening for a conversation. Alice replied,
rather shyly, "I—I hardly know, Sir, just at present—at least I know who
I was when I got up this morning, but I think I must have been changed
several times since that." (Carroll, 2008, p. 50)

Combined with the dream motif is the motif of subversion as Alice quickly learns that Wonderland will reliably frustrate her expectations and consistently challenge her understanding of the natural order in her world. She botches her multiplication tables, incorrectly recites poems she had learned in Wonderland, and finds that her lessons learned in real life no longer mean what she thought they did; in short Wonderland frustrates Alice's attempts to make meaning of her experiences logically where she can establish a relationship of cause and effect. When Alice uses the phrase "curious and curiouser" this suggests that both her experience of Wonderland and the language she uses to make meaning of it extends beyond convention and in this, her language reflects her newly discovered sense of limitless possibility (Dunn & McDonald, 2010).

The other characters in *Alice in Wonderland* were also subject to Freudian analysis; the dormouse's tendency to fall asleep is seen by Géza Roheim (1971) as a symptom of psychological withdrawal, while William Empson (1935) sees the Queen of Hearts as a symbol of uncontrolled animal passion.

Almost everything in Alice lends itself to symbolic interpretation; yet nothing clearly represents something specific. The garden, for example, on which Alice focuses much of her attention and effort to enter, could either be a symbolic reference to the Garden of Eden and its connotation to a desire to return to innocence (the pre-awakened state of the unconscious) as Alice attempts to hold onto the very child-like notions she must relinquish in order to mature; or alternatively in a more sexual reading of the tale could merely indicate unmet desire as she focuses much effort on her attempts to enter the garden, but is denied its pleasures (Goldschmidt, 1933).

A similarly sexual connotation was ascribed by some critics to the caterpillar's mushroom; some view the caterpillar's phallic shape as a symbol of sexual virility and see him as a sexual threat. The mushrooms have magic properties which Alice must consume to gain control over her fluctuating size, which represents the frustrations that accompany body image in puberty (Goldschmidt, 1933).

In *Through the Looking Glass*, Lewis Carroll explores the themes of reversal, reflection, and opposition. A looking glass is a mirror which offers a reflection as a reproduction, but with a difference from the real world. Mirrors reflect the opposite or backwards version of things, a theme consistently seen in *Through the Looking Glass*: the White Queen's finger bleeds before she pricks it; for Alice to get away from the look-ing glass house, she must walk towards it; and Alice and the Queen of Hearts have to run in order to stand still, as the order of cause and effect is reversed (Carroll, 1998).

The gender dynamic with particular reference to Freud's Eros/Thanatos archetypes

Insofar as the gender aspects in the Alice texts are concerned, Carina Garland (2008) suggested that they are malicious to the extent that they are spiteful attempts of the male author to suppress and control Alice as a result of his frustrated sexual desire for her. Carroll's anxieties regard-ing female sexuality and independence as well as his efforts to control these are expressed through the representations of food and appetite and the relationship of these to the feminine. Carolyn Sigler (1997) noted that as enjoyable as it is to walk with Alice through Wonderland, every now and then something disturbing almost awakens one from the dream.

She further noted that the Alice books have commonly been read as coming-of-age tales to do with the construction of identity and independence. Ulrich Knoepflmacher (1998) saw Alice as the subver-sive, active heroine and in his analysis in the gendered power struggle between Alice and the author, Alice wins. In citing the various instances surrounding food and hunger in the texts, Garland (2008) argued that this analysis is flawed in that Knoepflmacher failed to recognise the male repression and hatred of the power female sexuality represents in Carroll's attempts to quell the sexuality of his child heroine, Alice. Both Knoepflmacher and Sigler noted the difference in how Alice is por-trayed between Wonderland and its sequel, *Through the Looking Glass*, but Garland argued that these authors failed to fully appreciate the significance of the shift in how female sexuality is portrayed through Carroll's eyes.

She sees Carroll's portrayal of female sexuality as a destructive and frightening force but noted the differences in how the anxieties sur-rounding female sexuality are presented in that *Alice in Wonderland* is about possession, whereas *Through the Looking Glass* is about loss. Karoline Leach, in her biography of him in 1999, argues in line with Freudian analysis, that the male author is preoccupied sexually with his child heroine and that the difference in the portrayals of Alice in the two texts suggests that there is something the child heroine can offer that the adult Alice cannot; the girl represents the border between two states, and is presented as having a desire to transgress her embodied limit (Leach, 1999).

In support, Leach sheds light on Carroll's friendships with women, with him, an unmarried clergyman at times exerting a sexual, scandalous (for Victorian times) element on these relationships. But in her attempts to rescue Carroll from the overtones of paedophilia, Leach instead portrays him as a lecherous old man who hides his sexual desires and improprieties behind the veneer of an eccentric adult who preferred the company of children over that of adults (Garland, 2008). Garland asserts that the Alice texts, insofar as desire and sexuality are concerned, can best be understood through revisiting his portrayal of female figures as they relate to food, in particular with reference to Barbara Creed's (1993) notion of the vagina dentata (the vagina with teeth). The term, according to Creed, is indicative of the male fear of aggressive female sexuality and refers to a bestial, aggressive, destructive female sexuality (or with lesser emphasis on the sexual, in Jungian terms as the Death Mother), and reclaims Freud's theories around the phallus (Creed, 1993).

This can be seen in the Jabberwocky poem which represents the destruction of the vagina dentata, the aggressive female sexuality, where he gives Alice a phallic sword to kill the dragon which in this case, as the Red Queen's champion, is the very epitome of a representation of aggressive, predatory female sexual desire. The significance of this scene is that only by slaying the dragon with the phallic sword granted to Alice by her author, can she figuratively kill the mature and awakened sexuality that will become part of her as she approaches adulthood, and therefore stay as the idealised child Carroll wants her to be in Wonderland (Goldschmidt, 1933). Here the victory of the sword (recall, Alice was told by the caterpillar to let the sword do what it wants for it knows what it is doing) represents the victory of male desire over the mature female sexuality that was so repulsive to Carroll; the phallus overcame the vagina dentata according to Garland (2008).

But in *Through the Looking Glass*, the phallus fails, for this is a tale about loss of the female child to womanhood, expressed by Carroll as follows: "About nine or ten of my child's friendships get shipwrecked at the critical point where the stream and the river meet; the child friends once so affectionate become uninteresting acquaintances whom I have no wish to set eyes on again" (Goldschmidt, 1933, p. 331). Insofar as food is concerned, it is worth noting that all instances of Eros/Thanatos in *Through the Looking Glass* present as sado-masochistic, as illustrated in how food is personified in the poem about the Walrus and the Carpenter, where the male Walrus befriends the female child oysters and then eats them.

> *"It seems a shame" the Walrus said,*
> *"To play them such a trick.*
> *After we brought them out so far,*
> *And made them trot so quick!"*
> *The Carpenter said nothing but*
> *"The butter's spread too thick!"*
> *"I weep for you," the Walrus said:*
> *"I deeply sympathize."*
> *With sobs and tears he sorted out*
> *Those of the largest size,*
> *Holding in his pocket-handkerchief*
> *Before his streaming eyes …*
> *"Oh Oysters," said the Carpenter*
> *"You've had a pleasant run!*
> *Shall we be trotting home again?"*
> *But answer came there none –*
> *And this was scarcely odd, because*
> *They'd eaten every one."* (Carroll, 1998, pp. 235–236)

Here is a Walrus who all the while mourns the oysters he plans to eat, and as he does so, he "weeps for them", and a little girl Alice who remarks that she "likes the Walrus best … because he was a little sorry for the poor oysters" (Carroll, 1998, p. 236), and this theme of desiring while destroying continues throughout *Through the Looking Glass*. The rule of jam is the key philosophy of *Through the Looking Glass*: "Jam to-morrow, Jam yesterday, but never Jam to-day" (p. 247) and food is used to demonstrate the impossibility of achieving satisfaction on the other side of the mirror, as illustrated by the character of the White Knight said to be a caricature of Carroll himself.

It is the While Knight who introduces a pudding that he desires but admits can never exist, in emphasis of the Eros/Thanatos tension ever present in the text. Alice, upon entering the final chess square to become a queen (adult woman), has to leave the White Knight; he mourns her departure by singing a song of melancholy, "The Aged, Aged Man", which saddens Alice, but she finds she cannot cry, for at this point something in the exchange is irrevocably lost. So food connects the themes of loss, denial, and desire in *Through the Looking Glass*; in the same way the impossible pudding represents impossible desire and longing for the White Knight, so the talking pudding Alice encounters at the coronation feast becomes the final connection between Eros/Thanatos and the vagina dentata for the newly matured Alice—who now aggressively insists on eating the pudding at the feast despite being told it is impolite to eat food one has been introduced to and being reprimanded by the pudding itself. Her hunger, consistently denied through the text, now overwhelms her to the point where she is prepared to kill the talking pudding so that she can eat, and in this she becomes aligned to the fearsome adult women, the Red and White Queens, the Queen of Hearts and the Duchess and reaches the full queendom of the vagina dentata, for she will have her hunger satisfied and be denied no more.

CHAPTER 8

Synthesis of the major recurring themes

B y examining the five concepts, there were themes that became evident throughout the book, which will be summarised shortly.

Pre-agrarian humanity was food insecure. Unable to control the forces of nature and with agriculture in its very early phases of development, humanity looked to their gods to mediate their interaction with nature; much as the preconscious ego relates to the superego as an external locus of control in Freudian terms. Food was seen as a blessing from the gods and to access it, one had to be in communion with divinity. The depictions of the famously fat ancient goddesses, described earlier, is indicative of their divinity; for goddesses were not subject to the ravages of famine in a world of food insecurity. A special sign of provenance was in the themes of nectar and ambrosia (or manna and quails)—for not only was this the food of the gods, but they would bestow it on humanity as a special favour. Nectar and ambrosia represent what was particularly scarce in ancient times: energy dense foods, such as proteins (hence the hunting rituals and blood sacrifices) and sweet foods. These particular foods were reserved for special occasions and events of religious significance, and the well to do. To be fat was indicative of enjoying the favour of the gods more so than others;

for the ego in its unified state with the self wants to be favoured above others.

Similarly, the role of the gods was extended to mitigate other matters humans felt themselves unable to control, as seen in the tales of the banana goddess who mediated between husbands and their wives in lessening the imbalance in power relations characteristic of early patriarchal societies, and that of the gods' solution to the problem of Persephone who through their compromise could alternate between the realms of the dead and the living. In Jungian terms, the story of Persephone is about the gods and the fates (the collective unconscious) mediating the interaction between the unconscious and the conscious that occurs in the human psyche, whereas the banana goddess is similar in that here the goddess (unconscious) maintains the balance between the anima and the animus through compensation. The ancient myths and symbols also illustrate that imbalance in the psyche is expressed as neurosis or pathology; to cure the neurosis or the pathology, the imbalance must be restored.

Ancient society can also be read as a metaphor; during this time, much of the scientific discoveries that enable humanity to control their environment in the present day did not exist as they were still buried in the domain of the unknown (a metaphor for the unconscious). Hence the proliferation of gods in the ancient world and superstition that prevailed both in ancient times and during the Dark Ages before the dawn of the Age of Reason brought about by the increase in scientific discoveries. The ancient civilisations differed from the Dark Ages in that this was the period of the feminine divine, the sacred female alongside the male divine. The gods of Olympus were both male and female, and so were the ancient Norse gods and the gods in other cultures of the time. In the temples of several cultures it was the high priestess who reigned in a position of supreme spiritual authority; during this era, there was a general balance of the male and female forces represented by the anima and animus.

Then came the Dark Ages, the period in which the patriarchal monotheistic religions dominated. In the Western world, the early Catholic Church started finding its place and the pagan gods were displaced, along with the feminine divine; for spirituality was now male dominated and the balance between the anima and animus was disturbed. The period is characterised by witch hunts, plague, and war as the animus dominated. It was during this period that the holy anorexics found their place, and in Jungian terms, it can broadly be seen as a physical manifestation of an unconscious balancing, by compensation. The Freudian reading is different, in that Catherine of Siena's anorexia is seen more as a controlling behaviour and a reaction to the personal trauma, a response to the loss of her siblings, but the theme of female reaction to male dominance, that is, the imbalance between the anima and animus, remains.

While the gods of ancient times bestowed food as blessings onto humanity, there were limits; some foods were reserved for the gods. The golden apples in the garden of Hesperides, and the fruit of the Tree of Life in the Garden of Eden were forbidden to man, and to seek them would invoke the anger of the pantheistic gods or the biblical God. This illustrates another theme in the preconscious state: that the gods derived their ability to mediate between man and nature from the possession of privileged knowledge in the unconscious domain. This knowledge is represented by the forbidden fruits, and should humanity steal them, by entering the unconscious to decode its hidden contents and make it conscious, the journey of transformation follows. Once individuation is completed in Jungian terms, or the trauma buried in the psyche is made conscious in Freudian terms, the unconscious ceases to be unknown and can be controlled going forward, and the need for the gods to mediate between the conscious and unconscious worlds disappears. The gods then lose their standing.

Broadly speaking, the scientific discoveries that came with the Age of Reason also birthed the material universe, and religion and spirituality retreated into the background; for, able to control his world, man had no further need for the gods. The motif continues in the various stories painting dire consequences for those who dare anyway to eat the food reserved for the gods, for the gods will not go quietly and without resistance; this resistance must be overcome, and it is here where the Hero's Journey finds its place. Similarly, religious food taboos and dietary rules demonstrate adherence and unity with the gods; food is still consumed in communion with the gods. Many of these restrictions persist to the present day in the form of Kosher, Halal, and Hindu vegetarianism, amongst others. To break these rules is to break one's communion with the Divine. Here emerges another theme illustrated by metaphor: ritual encourages conformity, compliance, replicability, and discourages the disruptive and innovative thinking that leads to the exploration of the unknown.

Metaphorically these serve to contain the psyche in its conscious ego state. It is only when the psyche is traumatised and disrupted that this paradigm is overwhelmed and the Hero's Journey into the unconscious begins. The threat of Tantalus who was condemned to suffer through eternity for stealing the food of the gods, was meant to discourage Odysseus from entering the Garden of Hesperides in search of the golden apples. Christians are still reminded that eating from the forbidden tree is still the original sin that led to the fall of mankind, henceforth doomed to be born in sin. But by participating in the ritual of the Sacrament, or Holy Communion in which the bread represents the body of Christ and the wine his blood, eternal salvation could be found.

Eating the food of the gods had consequences beyond the ire of the gods; as a metaphor for the journey into the unconscious, the hero returns from his or her journey irrevocably changed. After Adam and Eve ate the fruit, they were banished from the Garden of Eden (the symbol of their naïveté or preconscious state), and they could never return. For in the Garden they did not realise they were naked, they subsisted on food provided by God, and both were created by God. They had dominion over the entire creation, but not over themselves. This illustrates the preconscious stage where the ego thinks it is in control and does not understand how the unknown in the unconscious is influencing the conscious behaviour.

Following the fall of mankind (similar to the fall of Alice into the rabbit hole) into the unconscious, Adam and Eve realise they are naked and to cover their nakedness, required the spilling of blood, the first sacrifice to God (now representing the unconscious) by killing animals (representing the ego which Adam and Eve had dominion over) to get the skin to cover them. Lewis Carroll's Alice had to slay the Jabberwocky (ego, also representative of the Death Mother archetype as the Queen of Hearts's champion), but was cautioned by the caterpillar (symbol of transformation) to let the sword (the unconscious) do what it wants as it knows what to do. It is the sword the Jabberwocky greets when meeting Alice (the hero) in the battle, not the insignificant sword bearer (the ego acting in the conscious). For the Hero's Journey of Campbell and Kudler (2004) demands that the infinitely more powerful unconscious be recognised and honoured; but doing so places the ego in great danger. To achieve the unified and conscious self requires growth and sacrifice; the slaying of dragons and Jabberwockys and the burning of witches as we face the shadow and transform the archetype of the Death Mother; for the Hero's Journey into the unconscious is not without consequence.

Adam and Eve now had the power of death and life, but that power meant they had to leave the Garden, the symbol of their preconscious state, as now they were able to control their destiny. Adam and Eve would now have to work the land to produce their own food from the sweat of their brow, and bear children in sorrow (give life). This is the transformed state of individuation. In Freudian terms, to unearth the trauma from the unconscious means one has to live with it in the conscious.

> Aniela Jaffé points out that in religious language an image of a God who seeks man just as much He is sought by man [sic]. God seeks the individual in order to realise himself in his soul and his life. Expressed psychologically: the self requires the ego-personality in order to manifest itself; the ego-personality requires the self as the origin of its life and its fate. In religious language, this means "God needs man, just as man needs God." (Jaffé, 1989, pp. 17–18)

These sentiments were echoed by Jung in writing to Erich Neumann, "God is a contradiction in terms; therefore, he needs man to be made One … God is an ailment man has to cure" (Jaffé, 1989, p. 99).

During Victorian times food production was more successful and trade became entrenched, allowing for relative food security. But the economic inequality of the day also excluded the masses from this bounty, and the overriding concern of the age was malnutrition and hunger. In this world where scientific discoveries were the order of the day and as the first industrial revolution took hold, divine favour as a symbol of what is uncontrollable to the ego started being replaced by socio-economic class, for this was the height of Newton's material universe. In this world of matter there was no place for ego, and class was the dynamic that explained why the majority had very little control over the quality of their lives.

As the problem of class remained unresolved through much of this era, God and religion still provided the imperative to restore balance; the abolition of slavery and the early works of charity were inspired by not only the noblesse oblige of the upper classes, but by their sense of piety. For the underclasses, the remedy was revolution to overthrow the social order which they perceived as oppressive. The popularity of religion waned as a concept associated with the upper classes; for the masses, divinity failed in its mediating role and as a balancing force in the social order. This is the ego's response to imbalance: the struggle to achieve the outward balance rooted in a conscious of separateness. This theme is echoed in the motif of gender in which the body shaming of women in the industrial age was explained by Naomi Wolf in 1991. The motif serves to illustrate the imbalance between the male animus and the female anima on a societal level as it presents as the battle of the sexes. When women entered the workforce, their reliance on men diminished and they became financially independent, diminishing the traditional male power base, and further threatening the male dominated social order by women demanding rights and access to roles in society traditionally reserved for men. In many ways, the feminist movement came as a conscious and ego-based response to imbalance, for patriarchy, unmitigated by a benign banana god, resulted in the repression of women and as such existed in a state of imbalance.

As this imbalance still persists and cannot be resolved in the ego state, the conscious balancing act of feminism is met with the counter-responses of discrimination and body shaming of women, as Naomi Wolf argues. Similarly, the development of agriculture and food production on an industrial scale overcame the scarcity of the Victorian times, and went alongside the introduction of public welfare systems which provide income support to the poor and removed the obvious difference between rich and poor—now everyone could eat in abundance. But this came at a cost; industrial food production while plentiful is not nutritionally equal to the whole foods consumed in moderation by the well-heeled, and consequently it is consumed in excess by the poor. In this context obesity became the outward manifestation of imbalance and because those better off are uncomfortable with what it represents and fear the consequences to their own class, the obese are shamed into submission, as Richard Klein (1996) and Paul Campos (2004) argue.

The understanding arising from advances in quantum physics allows for the collective unconscious from which the conscious world emanates, as the non-personal part of the psyche. It is a realm of archetypes which appear spontaneously in our consciousness, influencing not only our perception, thinking, and imagination, but also manifesting as physical matter as illustrated by contributions in the field of bioelectronics. In this context, Marion Woodman's theory of obesity based on cellular behaviour and genetic determinants finds its place, as she illustrates in 1980 by applying Jung's word association tests. High BMI people think very differently from others and these unconscious thoughts as wave forms exist in a state of potentiality where they can manifest in the physical world as matter—in this case genes and fat cells.

Woodman's contribution provides an illustration of how molecules are guided in their actions by the wave forms of their quantum states; and these quantum states are inner images— symbols, metaphors, and archetypes. These inner images control (as evidenced by quantum theory) all the processes in the universe, and as such translate in evolutionary terms. Biological evolution appears in the quantum world not as an adaptation of species to their environment, but as the adaptation of minds to increasingly complex forms—archetypes—which exist as wave states in cosmic potentiality. The same is true for the evolution of social systems and its structures of coherence and power including class, gender, religion, and the like.

It is when we reach into the collective unconsciousness to the archetypes that exist in their wave state as complex forms in the cosmic realm and actualise their virtual forms, that we are able to sustain life and give meaning to it. Ancient concepts embedded in these archetypes constantly re-emerge in our thinking; but they do so in an evolving manner. For example, Plato claimed that true reality resides in a realm of ideas which is outside the visible world. The concept is similar to the idea postulated by quantum theory that the empirical world actualises out of quantum forms existing in a state of potentiality in a cosmic realm, or as Jung's collective unconscious and archetypes. Jung wrote that the collective unconsciousness is:

> a boundless expanse full of unprecedented uncertainty, with apparently no inside and no outside, no above and no below, no here and no there, no mine and no thine, no good and no bad ... where I am indivisibly this and that; where I experience the other in myself and the other-than-myself experiences me ... There I am utterly one with the world, so much a part of it that I forget all too easily who I really am. (Jung, 1960, p. 21)

Because "they have never been in consciousness before" (Jung, 1960, p. 42) the archetypes exist in a state of potentiality in the non-empirical realm of the collective unconscious. Therefore, the birth of a conscious self comes from this realm of non-empirical forms through transcendence and individuation in the same way as the birth of the empirical, visible world of matter comes from a non-empirical realm of virtual states.

CHAPTER 9

A few last words on the recurring themes and concepts ...

In presenting the psychoanalytic framework, the association between obesity and the psychological structure of the person suffering was constructed. The recurrent themes occurring in both the Freudian and Jungian approaches suggest a relationship between personal traumas, depression (melancholia in Freudian terms), and loss, and suggest that obesity represents the attempt to fill a void that goes beyond food. This observation goes some way towards explaining why people who lose substantial amounts of weight, tend to relapse in 98% of the reported cases.

Obesity is a symptom of repetitive destructive eating patterns and the addiction to the repetitive cycle of weight gain and loss. The starting point for the design of a treatment model which integrates the insights offered by the psychoanalytic school would have to be based on the recognition of the mental suffering and the underlying trauma that gives rise to it. This requires a therapy that would focus on ways of dealing with the emptiness of one's existence—that void which the obese person is attempting to fill with food. The themes emerging from the literature suggest the possibility of a correlation between obesity and psychological suffering; in most cases, these two factors coexist.

When obese patients fail to adhere to the current treatment range of disorders of orality, it is an indication to involve them in their own symptomology; the very term obesity constitutes a structured phenomenon in language. However, on another level, it is also an enjoyment/ jouissance that captures the patient and leaves him or her in a state of suspension, for it is the state of complete suffering, both physical and mental that enslaves the obese patient. In this context, obesity is more than a mere somatisation, a psychosomatic disorder or a disease. Seen from the psychoanalytic perspective, obesity is a complex and unique disposition of the patient to become human (the individuated and reintegrated Self). The journey of individuation is dependent on the psychological structure of the person as it exists prior to, and during the individuation process. One of the recurring responses to episodes of binge eating noted in the second chapter of this book is depression, and similarly as Campos, Klein, and Wolf noted—prejudice against obesity is one of the most socially validated forms of prejudice. Obesity is often associated with moral weakness, lack of willpower, and a general sense of shamelessness on the part of the obese person; and frequently a total detachment between the patient as a human being and the symptom in the care environment occurs.

The body is treated only as a living organism and as part of the empirical reality of nature; medicine, dietetics, and biokinetics take care of it, requiring an imposed silence on the deepest meanings of the patient as if they are living in a body without a narrative. When combined with the behavioural and cognitive type approaches, a further layer of disembodied intellect is added. This results in the patient's subjectivity being progressively excluded from carrying any implication in relation to the process of getting sick, for the differentiation between the representation of the body in its physical form and the instinctual body which is the *real* body, which is situated beyond the representational body, is lost, and the real body is left untreated. This theme emerges when considering the Jungian contribution through the lens offered by quantum physics.

The instinctual body—as a category—distinguishes itself from the symbolic and biological bodies without excluding them; thus, the process of body transformation cannot be decoupled from the narrative of the body, and consequently the body investigated by psychoanalysis is very different from the body investigated by medicine, for this is a body that as a living organism, a collection of flesh, organs, and adipose tissue, is also a body that speaks.

Medicine is called upon to cure obesity as a disease, a disease that has psychological causes originating in the unconscious. The emergent theme illustrated by the literature calls attention to the necessity to articulate each one of the symptoms in the context of the narrative discourse produced by the body and the meaning of the different subjective experiences of the patient.

The information presented in this book suggests that the continued denial of the transcendent aspects of people's nature is what gives rise to the serious problems that are experienced in physical and mental health, of which the rising obesity epidemic is one such example. Therefore, the author concludes that to attempt to treat the incidence of obesity on the level of the conscious (as the behavioural and cognitive approaches suggest) and the physical (the dietetic, medical, and exercise approaches) will not yield satisfactory long-term results and this is what explains the almost universal relapse of 98% of obese patients who have achieved substantive weight loss, with the long-term success rate being less than two per cent.

A core theme that emerges in the literature pertaining to the underlying contributors of obesity, is that of trauma and loss. Psychoanalysis has focused extensively on the occurrence of psychic traumas at the source of neurosis. In the Freudian treatment of these themes, the theory of seduction (neurotica) presents a model that starts with excessive excitement which, if not relieved, becomes associated with an event, what Freud described as "après-coup", a belated attribution of traumatic memories which will become repressed. Traumatic events become connected to the original ghosts in the individual psyche and the afferent repressed anxiety. Applied to Freud's theory of infant sexuality, these would become the fears of castration, seduction, the primal scene, and the Oedipus and Electra complexes. In this context, trauma is associated with the strength of the sexual drive or libido in the psychological structure of the individual, at which point trauma becomes a breach in excitement resulting in a situation in which the ego is aggressively confronted with a reality of which it cannot make sense and to which it cannot attribute qualities.

This is the theme illustrated in the reading of the holy anorexic Catherine of Siena and in the Freudian reading of Lewis Carroll in the Alice texts. As the psyche receives an excessive influx of detached excitations without representation (meaning and attribute), the characteristic excess of trauma is always sexual in nature in Freudian theory and abandonment is the prototypical traumatic situation.

The concept of abandonment relates to the infant, who is incapable of satisfying internal functions, is totally dependent on the care of others to initiate instinctual life, and is evident as an underlying concept in Hilde Bruch's contribution on obesity in childhood, which she associated with a lack of maternal nurture. Trauma in a broader context is also associated with commotion, a reaction to endogenous or exogenous excitation which modifies the self (autoplastic), while trauma is alloplastic in that it changes excitation. For this composition of the self to be possible, it would require a previous partial or complete destruction of the preceding Self, as illustrated in the analysis of the Freudian reading of *Alice in Wonderland* which takes the concept of trauma further than that of originating in seduction, as Freud initially proposed, to the broader interpretation of trauma originating from a violation of thought and affection. This could come either as a result of disqualification or by way of denying the affection any recognition.

This requires the development of a therapeutic approach in which the early traumas are placed among negative experiences with other people, for these traumas are connected with several non-responses of the environment (including those originating from stereotype and relating to gender and class as shown in the text) to the affective needs of the obese patient. It is these situations that conspire to have the obese patient experience the asphyxiation of their psychic lives as a kind of paralysis of thought and the ego, that are secondary to the open wounds. The result of this process in the psyche is that of an egotistic rupture which once established brutally changes the relationship with the object (in this case the physical obese body and food).

If the relationship with the object becomes impossible, it becomes a narcissistic relationship in which the repressed unconscious is associated with the existence of affective states that are not integrated by subjectivity. This emptiness that results from the subjective fragmentation is the prerequisite for wanting something inside oneself and as such becomes the basis for the obese person's eating and learning of destructive eating patterns. If the emptiness took hold during an early life stage during which the obese patient was not mature enough to assign meaning to it, the patient unconsciously fears the horror of emptiness and will unconsciously defend against it at all costs, for example by organising controlled emptiness (not eating) or binge eating in an uncontrolled, compulsive manner.

It is the ego that organises the defence against the collapse of the organisation of the ego itself, and by making the unconscious conscious as the psychoanalytic frameworks suggests, the ego is always the structure being threatened and its defence will be established against a specific type of primal underlying agony—hence the often-absorbed inability of people with obesity to stick to the programme. For what is seen as a lack of willpower and self-discipline, may well be a primal ego defence, a key aspect to be considered in the development of a therapeutic model for obesity based on the psychoanalytic approach. For the ego's fear of collapse is the fear of a collapse that has already been experienced in some earlier stage of development and was not integrated satisfactorily into the structure of the ego.

The search for the feeling of fullness replaces the unbearable feelings of loss. The current approaches to the treatment of obesity all present the alternative to dependence achieved through the detachment of the object (food), but, as the repetitive patterns of binge eating in obese patients suggest, such an approach could lead to the unleashing of compulsive behaviour through which the patient tries to control the object (food). Faced with an unconscious trigger (such as a symbol), the patient will eat more and more, feeling fuller and fuller, but never quite full enough, and will eat again as the ego desperately tries to fill all the empty voids without fail. Obese patients are devoured by their own enjoyment and jouissance and in the end, despite repeated attempts to lose the weight, relapse as they resume their uncontrolled eating rituals. Feelings of self-condemnation and a sense of imprisonment inside their own obese bodies, as well as an emotion of powerlessness to break the destructive cycle of their uncontrolled eating, often follow these manic-like rituals, as depicted by Junia de Vilhena, Joana de Vilhena Novaes, and Carlos Rosa in 2012.

Freud (1940a) postulated the existence of an even more primal element than the psyche: the compulsion for repetition which precedes the principle of pleasure and its aim is to return to an inanimate stage which precedes life and stems from external disturbances. This compulsion to repetition is seen in the suicidal tendencies typical of severe depression, and in melancholia in the general sense—the lack of desire, the poverty of imaginative thought, and the repetitive and empty speech often observed in such patients. These are all manifestations of the strong presence of the death drive in the psychic life of the people concerned. Similarly, Freud described melancholia as the primitive stage of the anal-sadistic phase in which the patient abandons psychosexual reactions (jouissance) to the object (food), destroys it, and expels it; and this relationship is similar to that between the obese person and their food.

In this, Freud established a direct relationship between melancholia and disorders of orality, including obesity. Seen differently, melancholia is the result of a shadow of the ideal self (which is different from Jung's interpretation of the ideal self in that it is a construct created by the ego in this context). The ideal self is overvalued in the imagination and turns itself against the person, who is defenceless in psychological structure.

In the design of the recommended therapeutic model for the treatment of obesity, the question that arises then is how it would be possible to help the obese patient to elaborate the emptiness that results from the shadow of the ideal body. The ideal body is a social construct, created by the collective imagination and imposed on, and internalised by, people with obesity as a natural law of life, rather than something they can choose to pursue. While anorexia and bulimia are the incessant and pathological search for the ideal body (in the case of the holy anorexics, it was the pathological search for control over their lives and union with the Divine), obesity represents a relinquishment of this search in much the same way as the melancholic patient relinquishes the search for the ideal self. The most consistent manifestation of depressive mental disorders has a direct relation to the oral stage: a refusal to eat and the fear of starving to death (Vilhena, Novaes, & Rosa, 2012). Here eating replaces loving, and the depressed patient loses the ability to love while fearing death from love.

The Freudian conclusion is that in obese patients, libido had regressed to a more primitive stage of development: the oral stage, and that the more the genitals are replaced as the source of pleasure, the more people turn to oral eroticism, for unconsciously the melancholic patient will want to incorporate the object of his or her desire by either devouring it or destroying it.

The recognition of the underlying trauma provides the obese patient with the initial trigger to commence the Hero's Journey for the question the obese person to ask is, "In which mirror did I lose my face?" For existing is to present one's image to another; when something is not seen, it does not exist and is to be perceived. and being is being something to someone.

This first moment of critical reflection is explored in the fairy tale as an expression of the human psyche in Jungian analysis. While the archetypes have been subjected to conscious elaboration by the time they appear as fairy tales (Jung, 1959), the external events and characters of both myth and fairy tale can be seen as valid expressions of internal psychological dynamics. "In myths and fairy tales, as in dreams, the psyche tells its own story" (Jung, 1959, p. 40). If fairy tales reveal the psyche, the psyche arises as both an emotional crisis and an opportunity. The resource of consciousness is limited; life as the ego intended it is not working out and an impasse, a crisis arises either in the individual psyche or as the carrier of the collective consciousness. Marie-Louise Von Franz noted that consciousness is rarely capable of staying attuned to "all that is going on within and always tends to be too narrow, or to stay too long on one track ... In mythology, there are so often impotent or sickly or helpless and aged, rather than brilliant kings, for these represent the unadapted collective attitude" (Von Franz, 1972, p. 80).

The failure to remain in touch with the unconscious can precipitate the crisis that, for Jung, occurs when the sense of entitlement assumed by consciousness must give way to necessity. These crises become the catalysts for the development of a larger psychic centre, one that incorporates both consciousness and the unconscious that Jung calls the self (Jung, 1959, p. 315). Recent postmodern and particularly feminist critiques question the desire for wholeness central to traditional Jungian interpretation that the integrated self would represent. A traditional Jungian approach to fairy tales often defines masculine consciousness as the hero and feminine anima as the hero's counterpart (Jung, 1959). When the central figure of a fairy tale is female, Von Franz (1972) points out that she continues to represent the anima in masculine psychology, but female figures can also reflect the psyches of real women.

Where to from here?

The development of a therapeutic model for the treatment of obesity that combines the required dietary, medical, and physical interventions with a psychological intervention derived from the analytical and psychoanalytic approaches, seems inevitable. However, the model would have to be developed in a manner that not only integrates the physical and psychological elements of the model into a coherent therapeutic intervention, but also as one that is designed to overcome the excessive costs and time requirements associated with the psychoanalytic and analytical therapeutic models in their current form of delivery. Similarly, the model's development will be reliant on a multidisciplinary approach if its development is to result in a holistic but coherent model for the treatment of obesity.

The design task for an integrated model for the treatment of obesity may be thus articulated: to conceive of a model which investigates a superposition of a symbolic discourse as it appears in the sociocultural context, psychic and physical (somatic and environmental) objects. In building the model, the integration of the medical approach to obesity and the psychoanalytic approach must be achieved, but in addition the insights of the Freudian and Jungian schools of psychoanalysis must be integrated into a coherent continuum in a manner that reconciles the dialectic between the personal and collective unconscious. It is likely that such an eventual model will draw from the framework of intersectionality to allow for a coherent interpretation of an unlimited range of interaction of multiple variables.

Lastly …

The aim of the book was to explore the symbolic meaning of food, its influence on conscious behaviour, and how it developed through history and across cultures, in order to discover the root of obesity as seen through a psychoanalytic lens.

The folk tales and myths cited and applied throughout the text, from Marion Woodman's Othello to the twelve dancing princesses, Alice, Persephone, the original Hero's Journey told in the Epic of Gilgamesh and later echoed in Odysseus's twelve labours, are representations of the unconscious where the locus of psychoanalytical inquiry resides and where, given the point of departure of the book, it must lead, and presents a simple logical flow in the original thinking namely:

a. Obesity seems to have an underlying basis not addressed by the cognitive and behavioural approaches
b. This basis of obesity is likely to originate in the unconscious
c. The language of the unconscious is symbol and dream, and the unconscious is accessed through the archetypes
d. Therefore, to understand the unconscious contribution of pathological behaviour leading to obesity, the symbolic language of food must be understood, and similarly how these food symbols interact with the archetypes inherent in the individual psyche as well as the collective unconscious
e. As the unconscious is accessed through the archetypes, both symbol and archetype are expressed through culture and the collective

unconscious, and are represented in myth and folk tale (as products of the collective unconscious)

f. The way the archetypes manifest in the psyche helps to identify the underlying trauma

g. Obesity is thus the physical manifestation of an underlying trauma and is therefore not the disease, but the symptom, which then leads to the conclusion that

h. To resolve the obesity, the underlying trauma must be addressed.

A particular theme explored with specific relation to Jung's collective unconscious and Woodman's cellular theory was the recent advances in quantum physics and bioelectronics, which lends empirical support to Jung's notion of the collective unconscious and the manner in which it interacts with the personal unconscious. This provides some clarity and a framework within which to interpret one of the foundational tenets of the Jungian school.

The unconscious in relation to food and eating behaviour was explored, in a manner that allowed for the contents of the collective unconscious to be inferred through exploring the historical and cultural symbolic meaning attached to food, and found that in addition to the unconscious contribution of eating disorders (obesity), food as a social construct is imbued with a power and class dynamic, and continues to exert a powerful influence not only on how people become obese, but also on how obesity is treated and viewed in the treatment context.

Treatment approaches to obesity can thus be markedly improved by highlighting how the unconscious contents of the psyche serve to compromise conscious efforts to address the problem of obesity. And by incorporating the psychoanalytic approach to obesity, it will support the long-term success of weight loss intervention by addressing the underlying issues.

ACKNOWLEDGMENTS

I dedicate this book to Meike Wetsch, my soulmate and life companion, in celebration of our magic carpet ride of life together. Thank you for colouring in my life in all aspects and for always believing in me.

Also, a special thanks to my very dear friend and mentor Annelie Gresse for her limitless support and guidance, not only during the creation of this book, but also in life.

REFERENCES

Abraham, K. (1927). *Selected Papers on Psycho-Analysis.* D. Bryan & A. Strachey (Trans.). New York: Brunner/Mazel.

Adamski, A. (2011). Archetypes and the collective unconscious of Carl G. Jung in the light of quantum psychology. *NeuroQuantology, 9*(3): 563–571.

Ainsworth, M. S., & Bowlby, J. (1991). An ethological approach to personality development. *American Psychologist, 46*(4): 333.

Alice in Wonderland (2010). T. Burton, director. Walt Disney Studios Motion Pictures.

Allen, S. L. (2003). *In the Devil's Garden: A Sinful History of Forbidden Food.* Edinburgh, UK: Canongate.

Allison, D., & Heshka, S. (1993). Emotion and eating in obesity? A critical analysis. *International Journal of Eating Disorders, 13*(3): 289–295.

Ally McBeal (1997). D. E. Kelley (creator). Fox Broadcasting Company.

Andrade, A. M., Coutinho, S. R., Silva, M. N., Mata, J., Vieira, P. N., Minderico, C. S., Melanson, K. J., Baptista, F., Sardinha, L. B., & Teixeira, P. (2010). The effect of physical activity on weight loss is mediated by eating self-regulation. *Patient Education and Counseling, 79*(3): 320–326.

Andrews, T. (2000). *Nectar and Ambrosia: An Encyclopaedia of Food in World Mythology.* Santa Barbara, CA: ABC-CLIO.

Aquino, T., & McDermott, T. (1997). *Summa Theologiae: A Concise Translation*. London: Eyre and Spottiswoode.

Armstrong, K. (2005). *A Short History of Myth*. Toronto, Canada: Alfred A. Knopf.

Ashliman, D. L. (1998). *The Grimm Brothers' Children's and Household Tales (Fairy Tales)*. Princeton, NJ: Princeton University Press.

Atalayer, D., Gibson, C., Konopacka, A., & Geliebter, A. (2013). Ghrelin and eating disorders. *Progress in Neuro-Psychopharmacology and Biological Psychiatry, 40*: 70–82.

Averett, S. (2019). Obesity and labor market outcomes. *IZA World of Labor 2019: 32. doi: 10.15185/izawol.32.v2*

Bachelard, G. (1964). *The Poetics of Space*. Boston, MA: Beacon.

Banis, H. T., Varni, J. W., Wallander, J. L., & Korsch, B. (1988). Psychological and social adjustment of obese children and their families. *Child Care Health and Development, 14*: 157–173.

Banting, W. (1863). *Letter on Corpulence, addressed to the public ... with addenda*. London: Harrison & Sons.

Baranowski, T., Cullen, K. W., Nicklas, T., Thompson, D., & Baranowski, J. (2003). Are current health behavioural change models helpful in guiding prevention of weight gain efforts? *Obesity, 11*(S10): 24–43.

Barth, C., Bromiley, G. W., & Barth, M. C. (1991). *God with Us: A Theological Introduction to the Old Testament*. Detroit, MI: Wm. B. Eerdmans.

Bea, J. W., & Lohman, T. G. (2010). Long-term weight loss and chronic disease. *International Journal of Body Composition Research, 2010*(8): 21–28.

Bell, R. M. (1987). *Holy Anorexia*. Chicago, IL: University of Chicago Press.

Bettelheim, B. (1976). *The Uses of Enchantment: The Meaning and Importance of Fairy Tales*. New York: Vintage.

Birch, L. L. (1987). *The Acquisition of Food Acceptance Patterns in Children*. London: John Wiley & Sons.

Boakes, R. A., Popplewell, D. A., & Burton, M. J. (1987). *Eating Habits: Food, Physiology and Learned Behaviour*. New York: John Wiley & Sons.

Bosch, J., Stradmeijer, M., & Seidell, J. (2004). Psychosocial characteristics of obese children/youngsters and their families: implications for preventive and curative interventions. *Patient Education and Counselling, 55*(3): 353–362.

Bottigheimer, R. B. (2014). *Fairy Tales and Society: Illusion, Allusion, and Paradigm*. Philadelphia, PA: University of Pennsylvania Press.

Boutelle, K. N., Zucker, N., Peterson, C. B., Rydell, S., Carlson, J., & Harnack, L. J. (2014). An intervention based on Schachter's externality theory for overweight children: The Regulation of Cues pilot. *Journal of Paediatric Psychology, 39*(4): 405–417.

Bowlby, J. (1982). *Attachment and Loss*. 3 vols. New York: Basic Books.

Braet, C., & Crombez, G. (2003). Cognitive interference due to food cues in childhood obesity. *Journal of Clinical Child and Adolescent Psychology*, 32: 33–40.

Braet, C., & Van Strien, T. (1997). The DEBQ parent version. Assessment of emotional, external and restrained eating behaviour in nine to 12-year-old children. *Behaviour Research and Therapy*, 35: 863–873.

Bretherton, I. (1992). The origins of attachment theory: John Bowlby and Mary Ainsworth. *Developmental Psychology*, 28(5): 759.

Brewer, D. (1988). *Symbolic Stories: Traditional Narratives of Family Drama in English Literature*. Cambridge: Addison-Wesley Longman.

Brouwer, A. E. (2008). Globalization's contradictions: Geographies of discipline, destruction and transformation. D. Conway & N. Heynen (Eds). *Tijdschrift voor Economische en Sociale Geografie*, 99: 366–368.

Bruce-Mitford, M. (2008). *Signs and Symbols: An Illustrated Guide to Their Origins and Meanings*. London: Dorling Kindersley.

Bruch, H. (1941). Obesity in childhood and personality development. *American Journal of Orthopsychiatry*, 11: 467–474.

Bruch, H. (1961). Conceptual confusion in eating disorders. *Journal of Nervous and Mental Disease*, 133: 46–54.

Bruch, H. (1973). *Eating Disorders: Obesity, Anorexia Nervosa and the Person Within*. New York: Basic Books.

Bruch, H., & Touraine, G. (1940). Obesity in childhood: The family frame of obese children. *Psychosomatic Medicine*, 2(2): 141–206.

Brumberg, J. J. (1989). *Fasting Girls: The History of Anorexia Nervosa*. New York: Plume.

Bryant, R. A. (2001). Posttraumatic stress disorder and traumatic brain injury: can they co-exist? *Clinical Psychology Review*, 21: 931–948.

Bychowski, G. (1950). On neurotic obesity. *American Journal of Psychoanalysis*, 37: 301–319.

Bynum, C. W. (1987). *Holy Fest, Holy Fast: The Religious Significance of Food to Medieval Women*. Berkeley, CA: University of California Press.

Campbell, J. (1968). *The Masks of God: Creative Mythology*. New York: Viking.

Campbell, J., & Moyers, B. (1991). *The Power of Myth*. New York: Anchor Books.

Campbell, J. (2002). *Flight of the Wild Gander: Explorations in the Mythological Dimension: Select Essays, 1944–1968* (3rd edn.). Novato, CA: New World Library.

Campbell, J., & Kudler, D. (2004). *Pathways to Bliss: Mythology and Personal Transformation (Vol. 16)*. Novato, CA: New World Library.

Campos, P., Saguy, A., Ernsberger, P., Oliver, E., & Gaesser, G. (2006). The epidemiology of overweight and obesity: Public health crisis or moral panic? *International Journal of Epidemiology*, 2006(35): 55–60.

Campos, P. (2004). *The Obesity Myth: Why America's Obsession with Weight Is Hazardous to Your Health*. New York: Gotham.

Carroll, L. (1998). *Alice's Adventures in Wonderland and Through the Looking Glass and What Alice Found There*. New York: Oxford University Press.

Carroll, L. (2008). *The Complete Illustrated Lewis Carroll*. London: Wordsworth.

Cattell, R. B. (1963). Theory of fluid and crystallized intelligence: A critical experiment. *Journal of Educational Psychology*, 54(1): 1.

Chalmers, D. K., Bowyer, C. A., & Olenick, N. L. (1990). Problem drinking and obesity: A comparison in personality patterns and life-style. *International Journal of the Addictions*, 25(7): 803–817.

Cirlot, J. E. (1971). *A Dictionary of Symbols* (2nd edn.). New York: Philosophical Library.

Coulston, A. M. (1998). Obesity as an epidemic: Facing the challenge. *Journal of the Dietetic Association*, 98(10): S6–S8.

Craighead, L. W., & Allen, H. N. (1996). Appetite awareness training: A cognitive behavioural intervention for binge eating. *Cognitive and Behavioural Practice*, 1996(2): 249–270.

Cramer, P., & Steinwert, T. (1998). Thin is good, fat is bad: How early does it begin? *Journal of Applied Developmental Psychology*, 19(3): 429–451. *Personality and Social Psychology Bulletin*, 17(6): 606–611.

Crandall, C. S. (1994). Prejudice against fat people: ideology and self-interest. *Journal of Personality and Social Psychology*, 66(5): 882.

Creed, B. (1993). *The Monstrous-feminine: Film, Feminism, Psychoanalysis*. New York: Routledge.

Damms-Machado, A., Weser, G., & Bischoff, S. C. (2012). Micronutrient deficiency in obese subjects undergoing low calorie diet. *Nutrition journal*, 11(1): 1–10.

Dangerous Method, A (2011). D. Cronenberg (director). Montreal, Canada. Distributed by Entertainment One.

Davies, M. P. (1996). Review: The Portrayal of the Maturation Process of Girl Figures in Selected Tales of the Brothers Grimm. By Diann Rusch-Feja. Frankfurt, Germany: Peter Lang, 1995. *Journal of European Studies*, 26(4). doi:10.1177/004724419602600417.

De Castillejo, I. C. (1973). *Knowing Woman: A Feminine Psychology*. New York: Harper & Row.

D'Costa, K. (2013). *Eggs at Easter*. [Online.] Available at: https://blogs.scientificamerican.com/anthropology-in-practice/beyond-ishtar-the-tradition-of-eggs-at-easter/ (last accessed 21 April 2022).

De Lauzon, B., Romon, M., Deschamps, V., Lafay, L., Borys, J. M., Karlsson, J., & Charles, M. A. (2004). The Three-Factor Eating Questionnaire-R18 is able to distinguish among different eating patterns in a general population. *Journal of Nutrition*, 134(9): 2372–2380.

Diaz, V. A., Mainous, A. G., & Everett, C. J. (2005). The association between weight fluctuation and mortality: Results from a population-based cohort study. *Journal of Community Health, 30*(3): 153–165.

Dickens, C. (1837). *The Pickwick Papers.* London: Hazell, Watson & Viney, 1994.

Dieckman, H., Bettelheim, B., & Matthews, B. (1986). *Twice-told tales: The Psychological Use of Fairy Tales.* Asheville, NC: Chiron.

Dietz, W. H. (1983). Childhood obesity: susceptibility, cause and management. *Journal of Pediatrics, 103*: 676–686.

Dixson, A. F., & Dixson, B. J. (2011). Venus figurines of the European Palaeolithic: Symbols of fertility or attractiveness? *Journal of Anthropology, 2011*: 10–20. doi:10.1155/2011/569120.

Dombrowski, S. U., Knittle, K., Avenell, A., Araujo-Soares, V., & Sniehotta, F. F. (2014). Long term maintenance of weight loss with non-surgical interventions in obese adults: systematic review and meta-analyses of randomised controlled trials. *British Medical Journal, 348*: g2646.

Drenth, A. J. (2016). *Jung's Transcendent Function: Detachment, Symbols, & the Type Problem.* [Online.] Available at: https://personalityjunkie.com/12/jungs-transcendent-function-detachment-symbols-the-typological-problem/ (last accessed 21 April 2022).

Drieling, R. L., Rosas, L. G., Ma, J., & Stafford, R. S. (2014). Community resource utilization, psychosocial health, and sociodemographic factors associated with diet and physical activity among low-income obese Latino immigrants. *Journal of the Academy of Nutrition and Dietetics, 114*(2): 257–265.

Dunn, G. A., & McDonald, B. (2010). *Six Impossible Things Before Breakfast. Alice in Wonderland in Philosophy: Curiouser and Curiouser.* Hoboken, NJ: John Wiley & Sons.

Eddington, A. S. (1939). *The Philosophy of Physical Science.* New York: Macmillan.

Elder, G. R., & Cordic, D. D. (2009). *An American Jungian: In Honor of Edward F. Edinger.* Toronto, Canada: Inner City.

Elwell, F. (1996) *The Sociology of Max Weber* [Online.] Available at: https://academic.udayton.edu/RichardGhere/POL%20307/weber.htm#:~:text=Weber%20believed%20that%20the%20alienation,from%20the%20mode%20of%20production (last accessed 21 April 2022).

Ember, C. R., & Ember, M. (1988). *Anthropology.* Upper Saddle River, NJ: Prentice Hall.

Empson, W. (1935). *The Child as Swain. Aspects of Alice.* New York: Vanguard, 1971.

Evans, R. I., Jung, C. G., & Jones, E. (1964). *Conversations with Carl Jung and Reactions from Ernest Jones.* Princeton, NJ: D. Van Nostrand.

Faber, M. A., & Mayer, J. D. (2009). Resonance to archetypes in media: There's some accounting for taste. *Journal of Research in Personality*, 43(3): 307–322.

Fairburn, C. G., Wilson, G. T., & Schleimer, K. (1993). *Binge Eating: Nature, Assessment, and Treatment*. New York: Guilford.

Ferry, D. (1992). *Gilgamesh: A New Rendering in English Verse*. New York: Macmillan.

Ferster, C. B., Nurenberger, J. I., & Levitt, E. B. (1962). The control of eating. *Journal of Mathematics*, 1: 87–109.

Field, A. E., Austin, S. B., Taylor, C. B., Malspeis, S., Rockett, H. R., Gillman, M. W., & Colditz, G. A. (2003). Relation between dieting and weight change among preadolescents and adolescents. *Pedriatics*, 112: 900–906.

Fine, S., Haley, G., Gilbert, M., & Forth, A. (1993). Self-image as a predictor of outcome in adolescent major depressive disorder. *Journal of Child Psychology and Psychiatry*, 34: 1399–1407.

Flegal, K. M., Graubard, B. I., Williamson, D. F., & Gail, M. H. (2005). Excess deaths associated with underweight, overweight, and obesity. *Journal of the American Medical Association*, 2005(293): 1861–1867.

Forman, R. K. C. (1998). *The Innate Capacity: Mysticism, Psychology, and Philosophy*. Oxford: Oxford University Press.

Fouche, C. E. (2017). *Acquired Tastes: Virtue, Community, and Eating Ethically*. Gainesville, FL: University of Florida Press.

Frankl, V. E. (1984). *Man's Search for Meaning: An Introduction to Logotherapy*. New York: Simon & Schuster.

Freud, S. (1900a). *The Interpretation of Dreams*. New York: Macmillan, 1913.

Freud, S. (1940a). *An Outline of Psychoanalysis*. New York: W. W. Norton, 1949.

Frieze, I. H., Olson, J. E., & Good, D. C. (1990). Perceived and actual discrimination in the salaries of male and female managers. *Journal of Applied Social Psychology*, 20(1): 46–67.

Ganley, R. M. (1986). Epistemology, family patterns and psychosomatics: The case of obesity. *Family Process*, 25: 437–445.

Gardner, M. (1998). *The Annotated Alice*. New York: Random House.

Garland, C. (2008). Curious appetites: Food, desire, gender and subjectivity in Lewis Carroll's Alice texts. *The Lion and the Unicorn*, 32(1): 22–39.

Gilman, S. L. (2008). *Fat: A Cultural History of Obesity*. Cambridge: John Wiley & Sons.

Goffman, E. (1959). *The Presentation of Self in Everyday Life*. New York: Anchor.

Goldschmidt, A. M. (1933). *"Alice in Wonderland" Psycho-analysed*. Oxford: Basil Blackwell.

Goodman, M. (1980). *The Owl Was a Baker's Daughter: Obesity, Anorexia Nervosa, and the Repressed Feminine.* Toronto, Canada: Inner City.

Goodrick, G. K., & Foreyt, J. P. (1991). Why treatments for obesity don't last. *Journal of the American Dietetic Association, 91*: 1243–1247.

Goodwyn, E. (2013). Recurrent motifs as resonant attractor states in the narrative field: A testable model of archetype. *Journal of Analytical Psychology, 58*(3): 387–408.

Grebitus, C., Hartmann, M., & Reynolds, N. (2015). Global obesity study on drivers for weight reduction strategies. *Obesity Facts, 8*(1): 77–86.

Greenacre, P. (1955). *Swift and Carroll: A Psychoanalytic Study of Two Lives.* Madison, CT: International Universities Press.

Gregg, E. W., Gerzoff, R. B., Thompson, T. J., & Williamson, D. F. (2004). Trying to lose weight, losing weight, and 9-year mortality in overweight US adults with diabetes. *Diabetes Care, 27*(3): 657–662.

Grimm, J., & Grimm, W. (1884). *Household Tales.* London: George Bell.

Grimm, W., & Pacovska, K. (1812). *Hansel and Gretel.* Bristol, UK: Pook.

Gunstad, J., Paul, R. H., Spitznagel, M. B., Cohen, R. A., Williams, L. M., Kohn, M., & Gordon, E. (2006). Exposure to early life trauma is associated with adult obesity. *Psychiatry Research, 142*: 31–37.

Hafekost, K., Lawrence, D., Mitrou, F., O'Sullivan, T. A., & Zubrick, S. R. (2013). Tackling overweight and obesity: Does the public health message match the science? *BMC Medical Research Methodology, 11*(1): 41.

Harrist, A. W., Henry, C. S., Liu, C., & Morris, A. S. (2019). Family resilience: The power of rituals and routines in family adaptive systems. In: B. H. Fiese, M. Celano, K. Deater-Deckard, E. N. Jouriles, & M. A. Whisman (Eds.), *APA Handbook of Contemporary Family Psychology: Foundations, Methods, and Contemporary Issues Across the Lifespan* (pp. 223–239). Washington, DC: American Psychological Association.

Hawker, S., Soanes, C., & Waite, M. (2001). *The Oxford Dictionary, Thesaurus, and Word Power Guide.* Oxford: Oxford University Press.

Hebl, M. R., & Mannix, L. M. (2003). The weight of obesity in evaluating others: A mere proximity effect. *Personality and Social Psychology Bulletin, 29*(1): 28–38.

Hedley, A. A., Ogden, C. L., Johnson, C. L., Carroll, M. D., Curtin, L. R., & Flegal, K. M. (2004). Prevalence of overweight and obesity among US children, adolescents, and adults, 1999–2002. *Journal of the American Medical Association, 2004*(291): 2847–2850.

Heuscher, J. E. (1974). *A Psychiatric Study of Myths and Fairy Tales: Their Origin, Meaning, and Usefulness* (2nd edn.). Springfield, IL: Thomas.

Howitt, M. B., & DiTerlizzi, T. (2002). *The Spider and the Fly.* New York: Simon & Schuster.

Hoyme, J. B. (1988). The "abandoning impulse" in human parents. *The Lion and the Unicorn, 12*(2): 32–46.

Irwin, W., & Davis, R. B. (2009). *Alice in Wonderland and Philosophy: Curiouser and Curiouser (Vol. 20)*. Hoboken, NJ: John Wiley & Sons.

Jaffé, A. (1989). *Was C. G. Jung a Mystic? And Other Essays*. Einsiedeln, Switzerland: Daimon.

Johnson, S. L., & Birch, L. L. (1994). Parents' and children's adiposity and eating style. *Pediatrics, 94*: 653–661.

Jung, C. G. (1928). *Dream Analysis. Part 1*. London: Routledge.

Jung, C. G. (1934). *The Structure and Dynamics of the Psyche*. London: Routledge.

Jung, C. G. (1947). *On the Nature of the Psyche*. London: Ark Paperbacks.

Jung, C. G. (1948). The phenomenology of the spirit in fairy tales. In: *The Archetypes and the Collective Unconscious, 9 (Part 1)* (pp. 207–254). Princeton, NJ: Princeton University Press.

Jung, C. G. (1953). *Collected Works of C. G. Jung: Psychology and Alchemy*. Princeton, NJ: Princeton University Press.

Jung, C. G. (1959). The archetypes and the collective unconscious. *Collected Works (Vol. 9)*. Princeton, NJ: Princeton University Press.

Jung, C. G. (1960). *The Transcendent Function*. Kusnacht, Zurich: Jung Institute.

Jung, C. G. (1961). *Modern Man in Search of the Soul*. London: Routledge & Kegan Paul.

Jung, C. G. (1963). *Collected Works of C. G. Jung: Memories, Dreams and Reflections (Vol. 7)*. New York: Pantheon.

Jung, C. G. (1964). *Collected Works of C. G. Jung: Civilisation in Transition (Vol. 10)* Princeton, NJ: Princeton University Press.

Jung, C. G. (1969). *The Archetypes and the Collective Unconscious (Vol. 9)*. Princeton, NJ: Princeton University Press.

Jung, C. G. (1970). *Mysterium Coniunctionis (Vol. 14)*. Princeton, NJ: Princeton University Press.

Jung, C. G. (1982). *Aspects of the Feminine*. Princeton, NJ: Princeton University Press.

Jung, C. G., von Franz, M.-L., Henderson, J. L., Jacobi, J., & Jaffé, A. (1964). *Man and His Symbols*. London: Aldus.

Jung, C. G. (2012). *The undiscovered self. In The Undiscovered Self*. Princeton University Press.

Kafatos, M., & Nadeau, R. (1990). *The Conscious Universe*. New York: Springer.

Kaplan, R. M., & Saccuzzo, D. P. (2009). *Psychological Testing: Principles, Applications and Issues* (7th edn.). Belmont, CA: Wadsworth.

Karhunen, L., Lyly, M., Lapveteläinen, A., Kolehmainen, M., Laaksonen, D. E., Lähteenmäki, L., & Poutanen, K. (2012). Psychobehavioural factors are more strongly associated with successful weight management than predetermined satiety effect or other characteristics of diet. *Journal of Obesity, 2012.*

Karoly, P., & Kanfer, F. H. (1982). *Self-management and Behaviour Change: From Theory to Practice (Vol. 106).* Oxford: Pergamon.

Kats, S. H., & Weaver, W. W. (2013). *Encyclopedia of Food Culture.* New York: Charles Scribner's Sons.

Keränen, A. M., Savolainen, M. J., Reponen, A. H., Kujari, M. L., Lindeman, S. M., Bloigu, R. S., & Laitinen, J. H. (2009). The effect of eating behaviour on weight loss and maintenance during a lifestyle intervention. *Preventive Medicine, 49*(1): 32–38.

Kim, S., & Popkin, B. M. (2006). Commentary: Understanding the epidemiology of overweight and obesity—a real global public health concern. *International Journal of Epidemiology, 35*(1): 60–67.

Kirkham, T. C., & Tucci, S. A. (2006). Endocannabinoids in appetite control and the treatment of obesity. *CNS Neurological Disorders Drug Targets, 5:* 272–292.

Klein, D., Najman, J., Kohrman, A. F., & Munro, C. 1982. Patient characteristics that elicit negative responses from family physicians. *Journal of Family Practice, 14*(5): 881–888.

Klein, R. (1996). *Eat Fat.* New York : Pantheon.

Klein, S., Fontana, L., Young, V. L., Coggan, A. R., Kilo, C., Patterson, B. W., & Mohammed, B. S. (2004). Absence of an effect of liposuction on insulin action and risk factors for coronary heart disease. *New England Journal of Medicine, 350*(25): 2549–2557.

Knoepflmacher, U. C. (1998). *Ventures into Childland: Victorians, Fairy Tales, and Femininity.* Chicago, IL: University of Chicago Press.

Kvalem, I. I., Bergh, I., von Soest, T., Rosenvinge, J. H., Avantis Johnsen, T., Mala, T., & Martinsen, E. W. (2016). A comparison of behavioural and psychological characteristics of patients opting for surgical and conservative treatment for morbid obesity. *BMC Obesity, 3*(1): 6.

Landrigan, M. (2014). The bread rises like a voice: The intersection of food, gender, and place in the writing of Sheryl St. Germain. *ISLE: Interdisciplinary Studies in Literature & Environment, 21*(2): 298–314.

Lax, L. (2018). *Boost More than Your Metabolism with Apple Cider Vinegar.* [Online.] Available at: https://austinfitmagazine.com/January-2018/boost-more-than-your-metabolism-with-apple-cider-vinegar/#:~:text=In%20short%3A%20apple%20cider%20vinegar,it%20directly%20spikes%20your%20metabolism (last accessed 21 April 2022).

Leach, K. (1999). *In the Shadow of the Dreamchild: A New Understanding of Lewis Carroll.* London: Peter Owen.

Leach, M., & Fried, J. (1949). *Funk & Wagnalls Standard Dictionary of Folklore, Mythology, and Legend.* New York: Funk & Wagnalls.

Legenbauer, T., Petrak, F., de Zwaan, M., & Herpertz, S. (2011). Influence of depressive and eating disorders on short- and long-term course of weight after surgical and nonsurgical weight loss treatment. *Comprehensive Psychiatry, 52*(3): 301–311.

Lehner, E., & Lehner, J. (1971). *Devils, Demons, and Witchcraft: 244 Illustrations for Artists.* North Chelmsford, MA: Courier Corporation.

Lindenfeld, D. (2009). Jungian archetypes and the discourse of history. *Rethinking History, 13*(2): 217–223.

Lindstrom, M. (2008). *Buyology. How Everything We Believe about Why We Buy Is Wrong.* London: Random House Business.

Littleton, C. S. (2005). *Gods, Goddesses, and Mythology (Vol. 11).* Singapore: Marshall Cavendish.

Luna, A. (2014). Anima and animus: How to balance divine feminine/masculine. [Online.] Available at: https://lonerwolf.com/the-anima-and-animus/ (last accessed 12 April 2022).

Luthi, M. (1976). *Once Upon a Time: On the Nature of Fairy Tales.* Bloomington, IN: Indiana University Press.

Mario, J., Kast, V., & Riedel, M. (1992). *Witches, Ogres, and the Devil's Daughter: Encounters with Evil in Fairy Tales.* Boston, MA: Shambhala.

Markets and Markets (2016). Market research reports, marketing research company, business research by Markets and Markets. [Online.] Available at: http://marketsandmarkets.com (last accessed 12 April 2022).

Maroney, D., & Golub, S. (1992). Nurses' attitudes toward obese persons and certain ethnic groups. *Perceptual and Motor Skills, 75*(2): 387–391.

Marsh, P. (2004). Poverty and obesity. Social Issues Research Centre. [Online.] Available at: www.sirc.org (last accessed 12 April 2022).

Martin, L. (2016). Fantastical conversations with the other in the self: Dorothy L. Sayers (1893–1957) and her Peter Wimsey as animus. *University of Toronto Quarterly, 85*(2): 25–46.

Martinez, D., Turner, M., Pratt-Chapman, M., Kashima, K., Hargreaves, M., Dignan, M., & Hébert, J. (2016). The effect of changes in health beliefs among African-American and rural white church congregants enrolled in an obesity intervention: A qualitative evaluation. *Journal of Community Health, 41*(3): 518–525.

Maslow, A. H. (1943). A theory of human behaviour. *Psychological Review, 50*(4): 430–437.

Matsuo, T., Kato, Y., Murotake, Y., Kim, M. K., Unno, H., & Tanaka, K. (2010). An increase in high-density lipoprotein cholesterol after weight loss intervention is associated with long-term maintenance of reduced visceral abdominal fat. *International Journal of Obesity, 34*(12): 1742–1751.

Matthews, B. (1986). *The Herder Dictionary of Symbols: Symbols from Art, Archaeology, Mythology, Literature, and Religion.* Asheville, NC: Chiron.

McGuire, W. (1995). *The Freud/Jung Letters: Correspondence between Sigmund Freud and C. G. Jung.* London: Routledge.

McKenna, T. K. (1993). *Food of the Gods: The Search for the Original Tree of Knowledge: A Radical History of Plants, Drugs, and Human Evolution.* New York: Bantam.

Mendelson, B. K., & White D. R. (1985). Development of self-body-esteem in overweight youngsters. *Developmental Psychology, 21*: 90–96.

Mendelson, B. K., & White, D. R. (1995). Adolescents' weight, sex, and family functioning. *International Journal of Eating Disorders, 17*(1): 73–79.

Meyer, W., Moore, C., & Viljoen, H. (2008). *Personology: From Individual to Ecosystem.* Sandton, South Africa: Heinemann.

Miller, J. (2005). *The Impact of Locus of Control on Minority Students.* Menomonie, WI: University of Wisconsin-Stout.

Miller, J. C. (2004). *The Transcendent Function: Jung's Model of Psychological Growth through Dialogue with the Unconscious.* New York: State University of New York Press.

Mitchell, M. (1936). *Gone with the Wind.* New York: Simon & Schuster.

Mokdad, A. H., Ford, E. S., Bowman, B. A., Dietz, W. H., Vinicor, F., Bales, V. S., & Marks, J. S. (2003). Prevalence of obesity, diabetes, and obesity-related health risk factors, 2001. *Journal of the American Medical Association, 289*(1): 76–79.

Napoli, D. J. (1995). *The Magic Circle.* London: Penguin.

Neumann, E. (1955). *The Great Mother: An Analysis of the Archetype.* Princeton, NJ: Princeton University Press.

Neve, M. J., Morgan, P. J., & Collins, C. E. (2012). Behavioural factors related with successful weight loss 15 months post-enrolment in a commercial web-based weight-loss programme. *Public Health Nutrition, 15*(7): 1299–1309.

Nurkkala, M., Kaikkonen, K., Vanhala, M. L., Karhunen, L., Keränen, A. M., & Korpelainen, R. (2015). Lifestyle intervention has a beneficial effect on eating behaviour and long-term weight loss in obese adults. *Eating Behaviours, 18*: 179–185.

Ogden, J. (1966). *The Psychology of Eating: From Healthy to Disordered Behaviour.* Hoboken, NJ: John Wiley & Sons.

Olderr, S. (1986). *Symbolism: A Comprehensive Dictionary.* New York: McFarland.

Opie, I., & Tatem, M. (1989). *A Dictionary of Superstitions*. Oxford: Oxford University Press.

O'Reilly, G. A., Cook, L., Spruijt-Metz, D., & Black, D. S. (2014). Mindfulness-based interventions for obesity-related eating behaviours: a literature review. *Obesity Reviews, 15*(6): 453–461.

Pacanowski, C. R., Senso, M. M., Oriogun, K., Crain, A. L., & Sherwood, N. E. (2014). Binge eating behaviour and weight loss maintenance over a 2-year period. *Journal of Obesity, 2014.*

Pan, L., Sherry, B., Njai, R., & Blanck, H. M. (2012). Food insecurity is associated with obesity among US adults in 12 states. *Journal of the Academy of Nutrition and Dietetics, 112*(9): 1403–1409. https://doi.org/10.1016/j.jand.2012.06.011.

Parish, L. (1965). The Eysenck personality inventory by H. J. Eysenck & S. G. B. Eysenck. *British Journal of Educational Studies, 14*(1): 140.

Parsons, J. M. (2014). Cheese and chips out of styrofoam containers": An exploration of taste and cultural symbols of appropriate family foodways. *M/C Journal, 17*(1). https://doi.org/10.5204/mcj.766.

Petek, D., Kern, N., Kovač-Blaž, M., & Kersnik, J. (2011). Efficiency of community-based intervention programme on keeping lowered weight. *Slovenian Journal of Public Health, 50*(3): 160–168.

Phelps, E. A., & Le Doux, J. E. (2005). Contributions of the amygdala to emotion processing: From animal models to human behaviour. *Neuron, 48*: 175–187.

Pingitore, R., Dugoni, B. L., Tindale, R. S., & Spring, B. (1994). Bias against overweight job applicants in a simulated employment interview. *Journal of Applied Psychology, 79*(6): 909.

Polivy, J., & Herman, C. P. (1987). Diagnosis and treatment of normal eating. *Journal of Consulting and Clinical Psychology, 55*(5): 635.

Ponte, D. V., & Schäfer, L. (2013). Carl Gustav Jung, quantum physics and the spiritual mind: A mystical vision of the twenty-first century. *Behavioural Sciences, 3*(4): 601–618.

Popp, F. A., & Beloussov, L. (2003). *Biophotonics*. Dordrecht, the Netherlands: Kluwer Academic.

Puhl, R., & Brownell, K. D. (2001). Bias, discrimination, and obesity. *Obesity Research, 9*(12): 788–805.

Pyysiäinen, I. (2009). *Supernatural Agents*. Oxford: Oxford University Press.

Rejeski, W. J., Mihalko, S. L., Ambrosius, W. T., Bearon, L. B., & McClelland, J. W. (2011). Weight loss and self-regulatory eating efficacy in older adults: the cooperative lifestyle intervention program. *Journals of Gerontology Series B: Psychological Sciences and Social Sciences, 66*(3): 279–286.

Riebe, D., Blissmer, B., Greene, G., Caldwell, M., Ruggiero, L., Stillwell, K. M., & Nigg, C. R. (2005). Long-term maintenance of exercise and healthy eating behaviours in overweight adults. *Preventive Medicine*, 40(6): 769–778.

Roehling, M. V. (1999). Weight-based discrimination in employment: Psychological and legal aspects. *Personnel Psychology*, 52(4): 969–1016.

Roheim, G. (1971). *From Further Insights. Aspects of Alice*. New York: Vanguard.

Rölleke, H. (1988). New results of research on Grimms' fairy tales. In: J. M. McGlathery (Ed.), *The Brothers Grimm and Folktale* (pp. 101–111). Urbana, IL: University of Illinois Press.

Roman, L., & Roman, M. (2010). *Encyclopedia of Greek and Roman Mythology*. New York: Infobase.

Roser, M. (2014). Fertility Rate. *OurWorldInData.org*. [Online.] Available at: https://ourworldindata.org/fertility-rate (last accessed 12 April 2022).

Rowland, S. (2002). *Jung: A Feminist Revision*. Cambridge: Polity.

Schäfer, L. (2013). *Infinite Potential: What Quantum Physics Reveals about How We Should Live*. New York: Random House.

Schaverien, J. (2005). Art, dreams and active imagination: A post-Jungian approach to transference and the image. *Journal of Analytical Psychology*, 50(2): 127–153.

Schilder, P. (1971). *Psychoanalytic Remarks on Alice in Wonderland and Lewis Caroll. Aspects of Alice*. New York: Vanguard.

Schimmel, S. (1997). *The Seven Deadly Sins: Jewish, Christian, and Classical Reflections on Human Psychology*. New York: Oxford University Press.

Schlundt, D. G., Taylor, D., Hill, J. O., Sbrocco, T., Pope-Cordle, J., Kasser, T., & Arnold, D. (1991). A behavioural taxonomy of obese female participants in a weight loss program. *American Journal of Clinical Nutrition*, 1991(109): 1151–1158.

Schoemaker, C. G. (2004). A critical appraisal of the anorexia statistics in The Beauty Myth: Introducing Wolf's Overdo and Lie Factor (WOLF). *Eating Disorders*, 12(2): 97–102.

Shadraconis, S. (2013). Leaders and heroes: Modern day archetypes. *LUX: A Journal of Transdisciplinary Writing and Research from Claremont Graduate University*, 3(1): 15.

Sharp, D. (2001). *Digesting Jung: Food for the Journey*. Toronto, Canada: Inner City.

Sieff, D. (2009). Confronting death mother: an interview with Marion Woodman. *Spring: A Journal of Archetype and Culture*, 81: 177–199.

Sigler, C. (1997). *Alternative Alices: Visions and Revisions of Lewis Carroll's Alice Books: An Anthology*. Lexington, KY: University Press of Kentucky.

Skubal, S. M. (2002). *Word of Mouth: Food and Fiction after Freud*. London: Routledge.

Sobal, J., & Stunkard, A. J. (1989). Socioeconomic status and obesity: a review of the literature. *Psychological Bulletin*, 105(2): 260.

Soffiantini, G. (2020). Food insecurity and political instability during the Arab Spring. *Global Food Security, 26*: 100400.

Sommers, C. H. (1995). *Who Stole Feminism? How Women Have Betrayed Women.* New York: Simon & Schuster.

Spivak, A. P. (2014). The interpretive process: The power of "mere" words. *Journal of the American Psychoanalytic Association, 62*(6): 1063–1073.

Spurrell, E. B., Wilfley, D. E., Tanofsky, M. B., & Brownell, K. D. (1997). Age of onset for binge eating: Are there different pathways to binge eating? *International Journal of Eating Disorders, 21*: 55–65.

Staffieri, J. R. (1967). A study of social stereotype of body image in children. *Journal of Personality and Social Psychology, 7*(1): 101–104.

Stearns, P. N. (1997). *Fat History: Bodies and Beauty in the Modern West.* New York: New York University Press.

Stevens, J., Cai, J., Pamuk, E. R., Williamson, D. F., Thun, M. J., & Wood, J. L. (1998). The effect of age on the association between body-mass index and mortality. *New England Journal of Medicine, 338*(1): 1–7.

Stowell, P. (1983). We're all mad here. *Children's Literature Association Quarterly, 8*(2): 5–8.

Strauss, C. C., Smith, K., Frame, C., & Forehand, R. (1985). Personal and interpersonal characteristics associated with childhood obesity. *Journal of Paediatric Psychology, 10*: 337–343.

Stunkard, A. J., & Sobal, J. (1995). Psychosocial consequences of obesity. In: C. G. Fairburn & K. D. Brownell (Eds.), *Eating Disorders and Obesity: A Comprehensive Handbook* (pp. 417–421). New York: Guilford.

Svendsen, M., Rissanen, A., Richelsen, B., Rössner, S., Hansson, F., & Tonstad, S. (2008). Effect of Orlistat on eating behaviour among participants in a 3-year weight maintenance trial. *Obesity, 16*(2): 327–333.

Tatar, M. (1987). *The Hard Facts of the Grimms' Fairy Tales.* Princeton, NJ: Princeton University Press.

Tatar, M. (2002). *The Annotated Classic Fairy Tales.* New York: W. W. Norton.

Teufel, M., Stephan, K., Kowalski, A., Kasberger, S., Enck, P., Zipfel, S., & Giel, K. E. (2013). Impact of biofeedback on self-efficacy and stress reduction in obesity: A randomised controlled pilot study. *Applied Psychophysiology and Biofeedback, 38*(3): 177–184.

That Sugar Film (2015). D. Gameau (director). Australia: Madman Entertainment.

Thomas, J. (1989). *Inside the Wolf's Belly: Aspects of the Fairy Tale.* Sheffield, UK: Sheffield Academic Press.

Toole, J. K. (1980). *A Confederacy of Dunces.* New York: Grove, 1994.

Turner, V. (1975). Symbolic studies. *Annual Review of Anthropology, 4*(1): 145–161.

Vener, A. M., Krupka, L. R., & Gerard, R. J. (1982). Overweight/obese patients: An overview. *The Practitioner, 226*(1368): 1102–1109.

Vilhena, J. D., Novaes, J. D. V., & Rosa, C. M. (2012). Obesity: Listening beyond the fat cells. *Revista Latinoamericana de Psicopatologia Fundamental*, *15*(3): 718–731.

Von Franz, M.-L. (1972). *The Feminine in Fairytales*. Irving, TX: Spring.

Von Franz, M.-L., & Crossen, K. (1970). *The Interpretation of Fairy Tales*. Boston, MA: Shambhala.

Wallace, W. J., Sheslow, D., & Hassink, S. (1993). Obesity in children: a risk for depression. *Annals of the New York Academy of Sciences*, *699*(1): 301–303.

Watson, L. (1995). *Dark Nature: Natural History of Evil*. London: Hodder & Stoughton.

Wells, J. C. (2010). *The Evolutionary Biology of Human Body Fatness: Thrift and Control (Vol. 58)*. Cambridge: Cambridge University Press.

Westerterp-Plantenga, M. S., Kempen, K. P. G., & Saris, W. H. M. (1998). Determinants of weight maintenance in women after diet-induced weight reduction. *International Journal of Obesity & Related Metabolic Disorders*, *22*(1): 1–6.

Wilson, G. T. (1994). Behavioural treatment of obesity: Thirty years and counting. *Advances in Behaviour Research and Therapy*, *16*: 31–75.

Wolf, N. (1991). *The Beauty Myth: How Images of Beauty Are Used against Women*. New York: Morrow.

Wolkstein, D., & Kramer, S. N. (1983). *Inanna, Queen of Heaven and Earth: Her Stories and Hymns from Summer*. New York: Harper & Row.

Woodman, M. (1980). *The Owl Was a Baker's Daughter: Obesity, Anorexia Nervosa and the Repressed Feminine*. Toronto, Canada: Inner City.

Woolf, V. A. (1957). *Room of One's Own*. New York: Harcourt, Brace and World.

Woolverton, L., & Burton, T. (2010). *Alice in Wonderland* [the movie]. Burbank, CA: Walt Disney Pictures.

World Health Organization (2003). Diet, nutrition and the prevention of chronic diseases. Report of a joint WHO/FAO expert consultation. Geneva, Switzerland: World Health Organization.

World Health Organization (2015). Strategy on diet, physical activity and health (Fact sheet No. 312). [Online.] Available at: http://who.int/mediacentre/factsheets/fs311/en/ (last accessed 12 April 2022).

Yeh, M., Chu, N., Hsu, M. F., Hsu, C., & Chung, Y. (2015). Acupoint stimulation on weight reduction for obesity: A randomized sham-controlled study. *Western Journal of Nursing Research*, *37*(12): 1517–1530.

Zipes, J. (1997). *Happily, Ever After: Fairy Tales, Children and the Culture Industry*. New York: Routledge.

Despite all efforts that have been made to mention all authors, the references of some authors may have been omitted to enhance the reading quality of the book, as the rework of the book is not intended to be academic. If any authors have been excluded in this book, please contact me in order to include the references in the next print.

INDEX

CPSIA information can be obtained
at www.ICGtesting.com
Printed in the USA
JSHW022217151022
31677JS00003B/4